Twelve Weeks to a Bette

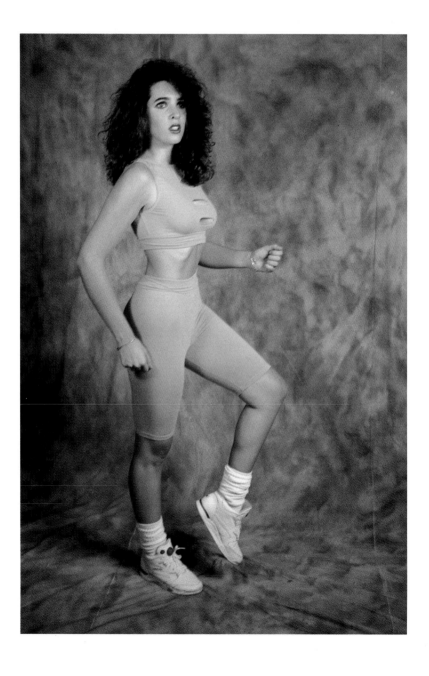

Twelve Weeks to a Better Body for Women

Ronald S. Laura and Kenneth R. Dutton

ALLEN & UNWIN

To my daughter Helene for her enthusiasm and dedication to health and fitness, and for her contribution to the evolution of the Twelve Week Matrix program.

Ronald S. Laura

First published in 1994

Allen & Unwin Pty Ltd
9 Atchison Street, St Leonards, NSW 2065 Australia

National Library of Australia
Cataloguing-in-Publication entry:

Laura, R. S. (Ronald S.)
  Twelve weeks to a better body for women.

  ISBN 1 86373 483 X.

  1. Physical fitness for women. 2. Self-care, Health.
  3. Weight training for women. 4. Women—Nutrition.
  I. Dutton, K. R. (Kenneth Raymond), 1938– . II. Title.
  III. Title: 12 weeks to a better body for women.

613.71

Set in 10/12 pt Garamond by DOCUPRO, Sydney
Printed by Kim Hup Lee Printing Co (Pte) Ltd, Singapore

10 9 8 7 6 5 4 3 2

The authors have great faith in this program but cannot take responsibility for injury caused to readers. As with any exercise program, it should be undertaken with care and with individuals working at their own pace. Seek your doctor's advice to ensure that you are in good health before embarking on this program.

Contents

Part I
Before you begin

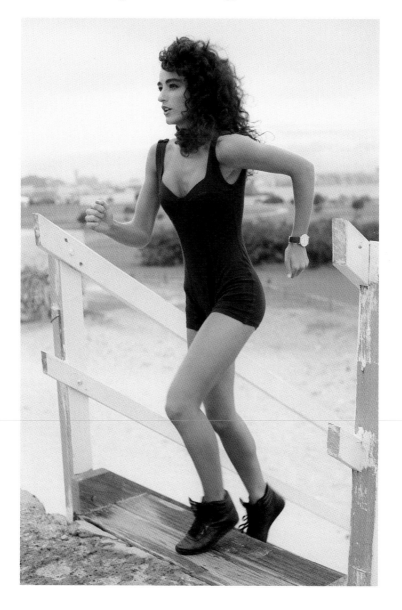

Let's be frank . . . most women want a better body

Many women nowadays are turning to exercise to develop a fit, healthy and active body—a body that says not just 'I care about how I look' but 'I care about who I am'.

This is not just a matter of outward appearance. It's a matter of looking after our body because we have value and importance as individuals. A body that we can be proud of enhances our personal confidence and gives us a more positive self-image.

We may not aim to develop a 'perfect' body (whatever that may be), but most of us will admit, if we're honest with ourselves, that we could improve on what we've got.

BETTER IN WHAT WAY?

When we talk of a 'better body', we tend to think immediately of our external appearance—that is, of a *better looking* body. This is fine as far as it goes—and there are few of us who don't want to enhance our physical attractiveness—but it doesn't go far enough. A better body is not just one that looks better, it is also a body that is fitter and healthier.

Fitness and health are often thought of as the same thing, but exercise physiologists usually distinguish between them. Fitness is generally associated with an efficiently functioning cardio-respiratory system—a heart, lungs and vascular system that maintains our capacity for sustained energy expenditure and has an important role in the avoidance of cardiovascular and respiratory disease, and thus helps in promoting longevity. Fitness also refers to a well-functioning muscular system, one that will help us avoid strain or injury to tendons and ligaments and even the skeletal system, especially the spine.

Health is a more general concept than fitness, and takes in a whole variety of lifestyle factors. It includes sensible diet, the avoidance of

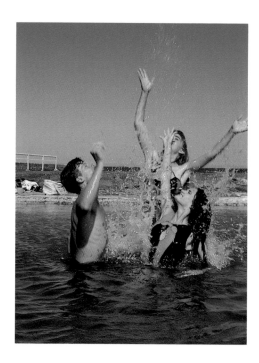

Healthy bodies for fun and fitness

smoking and excessive alcohol consumption, and the ability of the total organism to resist disease. While health and fitness are ultimately more important than looks, there is an organic relationship between them, such that a fit and healthy body will tend to look more physically attractive than one that is out of condition.

TOTAL HEALTH

Health is more than just a physical concept, however. We talk of 'mental health', and although this usually refers to freedom from the more devastating psychological diseases there is also a sense in which it is relevant to the general state of our body. A number of the more common psychological disorders which affect people in today's society have their roots in a poor, or even distorted, self-image which may be associated with how these people feel about their bodies.

Two of these disorders in particular—anorexia and bulimia—tend to affect women especially. In an obsessive quest for physical 'perfection', some people are led to go completely overboard, and literally to sacrifice both fitness and health (physical and mental) in pursuit of their impossible dream. Excessive dieting, 'pill-popping' and other harmful practices are adopted, which only heighten the sense of inadequacy and failure that led to their adoption. This is the very opposite of the 'better body' that this book is all about, and which it aims to help you achieve.

TODAY'S WOMAN AND HER BODY

The women's liberation movement has had a profound effect on how women tend to feel about their bodies. While some of the more radical of feminists have rejected any interest in 'looking good' as mere conformity to the values of a male-dominated society, most women have either refused or abandoned such extremism, seeing it as counterproductive and demeaning to women and the pride they should take in themselves and their bodies.

What has changed, and for the better, is modern women's *motivation* in looking after their bodies and enhancing their appearance. It is no longer because someone else dictates to them that this is how they 'must' look, but because this is how they choose to see themselves and to value themselves in their own eyes. If it has the added benefit of making them more attractive in the eyes of their friends, husband or loved one, so much the better, since it adds to their sense of empowerment and self-confidence.

With this change in attitude, there are signs that at least some women are developing a healthy scepticism about the so-called 'ideal' images presented to them in the popular media. The lanky, emaciated fashion model is no longer seen as the sole image of attractive femininity to which all women must aspire to conform. Whether women or men, nature has simply not endowed us all with the same physical attributes. Some of us are naturally short and thickset, others are built like a beanpole; others again seem to be too thin in some places and too thick in others. This is all part of life's rich variety, and it would be a depressing world for the vast majority of us if we could not feel good about ourselves simply because we do not naturally conform to a particular image.

The more sensible approach, as more and more women are coming to realise, is to make the best of what we've got—and to improve on it as much as we reasonably can.

THERE'S ALWAYS ROOM FOR IMPROVEMENT

Our natural frame (or skeleton) cannot be altered. But our body surface can be shaped and moulded to enhance our best features and downplay our worst. After all, the change in our appearance that happens naturally as we get out of condition and let our bodies 'go' is just such a process of remodelling, and usually in a direction we don't want.

What we can do, then, is to reverse the process by getting back into top condition. The method explained in this book will help you to do this by the most natural of means—the repeated movement of the body itself in a series of light exercises designed to restore its muscle tone and firm it up. At the same time, these exercises will improve your general fitness and help you get more enjoyment from life.

AS WE GET OLDER

Regrettably, the years take their toll on the body, and once we pass the age of 30 a decline in muscle tone starts to become apparent unless we take positive steps to do something about it.

Our fitness, too, begins to decline: for every decade past the age of 30 the capacity of the heart to pump blood decreases in the average person by 6–8 per cent. Our bones reach their maximum density at around the age of 30; from then on they slowly begin to lose mass, and we become more prone to degenerative joint disease. In the case of older women, osteoporosis or a marked loss of bone density becomes a more frequent problem.

The message may seem bleak, particularly when we think of the loss in skin elasticity, the decline in strength and co-ordination, skeletal disorders (such as osteoarthritis) and loss of memory—all of which become more of a problem the older we get.

THERE IS GOOD NEWS

But there *is* something we can do about it. Research studies have shown that those who exercise regularly can significantly retard the processes of ageing. Older athletes (aged 53–65 years), for example, have been shown to have oxygen uptakes 20 to 30 per cent higher than non-exercisers in their own age group, and only half the decline per decade which their non-exercising peers exhibit beyond the age of 25.

Osteoporosis, a loss of calcium from the bones which tends to affect post-menopausal women in particular, can also be retarded or even reversed by regular exercise. A Canadian study on the effects of supervised exercise (30 minutes per day, three times a week) on the bone density of a group of sedentary post-menopausal women showed that after one year bone density increased in the exercising group, while the control group of women who did little or no exercise showed no change.

The common misconception that as we grow older we need to exercise *less* should therefore be replaced by the understanding that in fact we need to exercise *more*.

EXERCISE IS THE KEY

Those who do currently exercise should not stop as they grow older. And even for those who have not undertaken regular exercise in their earlier years, the use of light weights in an exercise regime can produce beneficial results—from enhanced cardiovascular fitness and endurance to increased flexibility, better toned muscles and skin, and improved general health.

In addition to these physical consequences, the psychological outcomes they encourage are vitally important. As the body begins to improve in overall fitness, so mental attitudes tend to become more positive and exercisers begin to 'think younger'. Clinical studies have shown that vigorous exercise can reduce anxiety states for up to four hours after a workout, and are more effective than quiet rest in achieving this result.

You are never too old to start exercising, provided you warm up thoroughly and do not 'overdo' it. The exercises given in this book have been used by people of advanced age, including those in their 80s and even 90s! All of them have reported increased mobility and a more active interest in the world around them.

BEFORE YOU START

It is always a good idea to have a medical checkup before you begin a program of vigorous exercise, particularly if you have not done any systematic exercise previously, or—if you are older—have not done so in recent years. Especially if you have a history of heart, joint or muscle problems, a check with your doctor is strongly recommended.

Once you get the 'green light', you are ready to go. By all means set your sights on the visible goal you are aiming to achieve, but remember that it is still some way off. Don't be discouraged by the wait, but concentrate on the *process*: from your first exercise session onwards you are already developing a new concern for your body and a new awareness of your capabilities.

Even before the first visible results begin to appear, you have already changed: you have taken control of your body and begun to shape its future.

Weights? Me? No way!

I don't want to look 'muscly' . . . The answer is simple: you won't. Women often tend to shy away from resistance exercise (which is what 'weight training' really is) because of a fear that it will make them look more masculine or muscular. They are wrong.

They probably have in their minds images of 'women bodybuilders' or heavyweight female athletes (shotputters, discus-throwers and the like), who train in very special ways to build up their bulk and muscularity. Many of these women were, in any case, heavily built and muscular in the first place, and some even resort to dangerous drugs such as anabolic steroids to build up their 'abnormal' strength or appearance.

Instead of looking to these unusual cases, women should look more to the female sprinters, divers, gymnasts and other sportswomen who regularly use resistance training as part of their exercise regime. Here they will find plenty of lithe, athletic 'role models' who retain all their femininity and physical attractiveness.

WOMEN EXERCISERS LOOK FIRMER AND MORE ATTRACTIVE

Possibly because of endocrine differences between the sexes, women's response to resistance training is very different from that of men. Research by the US National Strength and Conditioning Association has shown that women who train with weights demonstrate a reduction in fat weight, an increase in lean weight, and either no change or only a slight increase in total body weight. In many cases they also show a decrease in lower body girth (that is a firming-up around the hips and buttocks).

If confirmation is needed, think of the many women film stars (and even professional models) who nowadays commonly exercise with light weights. In professions in which women rely on a 'trim, taut and terrific' figure to maintain an attractive and feminine appearance, the regular weight-exercise session has been found to be an indispensable aid in looking good for the camera.

CAN'T I JUST DO SOME AEROBICS?

Of course. Aerobics, like other forms of cardiovascular exercise, will help maintain your general fitness and keep your circulation system in good shape. Together with other factors—sensible diet, not overeating or drinking to excess, not smoking and the like—it can be an important element of an overall healthy lifestyle. If you're overweight, out of condition or in your later years, you would do better to try (or at least to start with) the less intense exercise of 'low impact' aerobics. Jogging, too, may appeal to some, though if you are obese or out of shape it is probably not a sensible idea in view of the strain it can place on the joints and even on the heart. A much better and safer plan is to take up walking, aiming to cover 2 to 3 kilometres (or a mile and a half) every day at a comfortable speed and increasing your distance (not your speed) as your fitness improves.

Keep in mind, though, that these cardiovascular benefits are not the only aim of your exercise program. Aerobic-type exercise certainly burns kilojoules (or calories) while you are doing it and for a short time—perhaps 20–40 minutes—afterwards. Resistance training, however, maintains this kilojoule-burning (known as 'elevated metabolism') for at least an hour after the workout. In the case of certain types of weight training, like the kind you will find in this book, the elevated metabolism can continue for several hours or even days.

People who concentrate exclusively on aerobic exercise may also neglect the need to build up and maintain their strength, particularly upper-body strength—in the arms, chest and back, for example. And strength is an important component of general fitness. Studies undertaken with retirees (both male and female) in Boston showed that two weight workouts per week not only improved muscle tone—as you would expect—but also had a beneficial effect on joint mobilisation and bone density.

BUILDING LEAN TISSUE

In addition, you are building muscle tissue. (Don't take fright at the thought—the effect will show up in improved muscle tone rather than in bulging biceps!) Muscle tissue is referred to as 'metabolically active'—that is, it actually consumes kilojoules simply in order to maintain itself.

This is where muscle differs from fat. To sustain muscle cells requires considerable energy, while to sustain fat cells requires virtually none. The fatter we are, then, the less energy we need to maintain the same body state; the more lean muscle we carry, the more energy we need in order to maintain it. The 'energy' comes in the form of the kilojoules we burn, so if we increase our muscle we burn up more kilojoules even if our diet remains the same.

BURNING AWAY THE UNWANTED KILOS

A single kilogram of muscle, simply in order to maintain itself, requires 60–90 kilojoules per day. So, if you are replacing fat by muscle tissue, you will be burning away the kilojoules even if your body weight remains the same. (Muscle is heavier than fat, which is why your body weight may not actually decrease for a while.)

If you have already been doing aerobics and can find the time to keep doing it in conjunction with your resistance training, by all means do so. If not, you will still find that the exercises in this book have a beneficial effect on the cardiovascular system, as well as burning away the fat even more efficiently.

WHAT ABOUT DIET?

Of course, appropriate diet is vitally important. Whilst a small percentage of women in our society are underweight and need to pay more attention to an intake of sustaining and healthy food as part of their fitness regime, a far greater number have the opposite problem. It has been estimated that up to one-third of Australian women (and up to one-half of Australian men) are overweight.

This, again, is not simply a matter of personal appearance. Obesity increases the risk of hypertension, respiratory problems, gallstones and numerous other health hazards, quite apart from overloading the joints and increasing the risk of osteoarthritis.

The enormous popularity of 'fad' diets (including so-called 'crash' diets) and weight-loss centres shows just how many people in our society are seeking to shed excess weight. Part of the problem with dieting is that much of the loss tends to be by way of water and lean

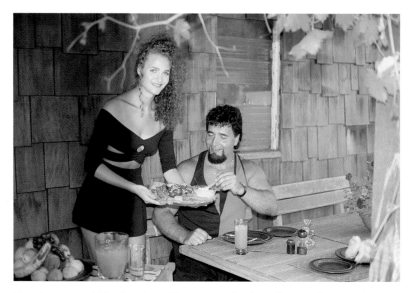

Ron Laura and his daughter Sharon get the benefit out of raw and whole foods.

muscle tissue rather than fat. In one recent study of dieters, 40 per cent of the weight loss achieved took the form of lean tissue.

On the other hand, exercise alone (without dietary modification) tends to have a rather slow effect in achieving weight loss, partly because the rise in energy expenditure is considerably less than the normal day's metabolic requirement—not to mention the fact that some people tend to feel like eating more when they begin to exercise! Moreover, people who are obese and unfit tire quickly during exercise and are thus limited in their ability to expend kilojoules.

The ideal combination for weight loss is a reduction in food intake along with a reasonably vigorous (but not overtaxing) exercise regime. The increased metabolic effect of exercise means that less of our energy intake is stored within the body, and there is an increase in the proportion of fat rather than lean muscle which is lost through our reduced dietary intake. In the study quoted above, when moderate exercise was added to diet the same amount of weight was lost but only 25 per cent of this was lean tissue (as distinct from 40 per cent with diet alone).

In summary, by combining your exercise regime with a sensible, long-term diet (not a 'crash' diet), you will ensure that you maximise your fat loss and minimise the loss of lean muscle tissue resulting

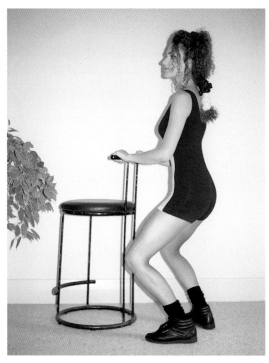

Sharon Laura
demonstrates how
items around the
house can provide all
the equipment you
need for a Matrix
workout.

from your reduced food intake. At the same time, the gains you make through your exercise will be entirely by way of new lean tissue and not fat. As your fitness improves, the intensity and vigour of your exercise regime will also increase, and with them your energy expenditure and weight control.

Further information on diet is provided in the appendix.

I'M TOO FAT IN SOME PLACES AND TOO SKINNY IN OTHERS

This is a common problem as we get older. Not only the proportion but also the distribution of body fat changes with age. Women often notice how the fat seems to have shifted, as they grow older, from their arms to their thighs and abdomen, leaving the skin of their upper arms hanging loosely.

This is where the double effect of weight exercise can be helpful. In addition to reducing body fat by burning up kilojoules, it restores muscle tone (and thus skin tone) to all those surface areas where the underlying muscles can be actively developed, keeping them firm and shapely rather than weak and sagging.

Remember what we said earlier: our bodies are in a constant state of transformation. While we cannot reverse the processes of ageing, we need to remember that some of the changes that take place as we grow older are due, not to age itself, but to changes in our lifestyle and our pattern of activity. Along with our dietary decisions, the amount and type of exercise we do are factors for change which are *within our control*: much of the 'redistribution' we observe in the shape of our bodies is wrongly attributed to the irreversible processes of ageing, and we overlook the extent to which the future of our bodies lies in our own hands.

BUT I CAN'T GET TO A GYM

Don't worry; you don't need to. The exercise program in this book has been designed to let you exercise at home. Naturally, if you *can* get to a gym you will find a wider range of exercise equipment and that will allow you a good deal more variety in the exercises you can do.

It may be that you do live reasonably close to a gym, but that you are reluctant to go there because you see it as an 'all-male' preserve. In that case, perhaps you haven't looked inside a gym lately—in most of them these days you will find plenty of women 'working out' with the men.

Nonetheless, we realise that some women simply do not have the time or the opportunity (or the money!) to enrol at a gym. Others again—at least when they are raw beginners—are just too embarrassed about how they look to feel confident about walking into a weight-room. (In this case, we hope that this book will improve your appearance—and your self-confidence—so that this will no longer be a problem.)

YOU CAN DO ALL THESE EXERCISES AT HOME

The program presented in this book is designed to be performed in your own home and requires a minimum of equipment. All you will need to begin with is a broomstick or a length of hollow pipe and a couple of light dumbbells (say 2–3 pounds—a kilogram or so) which can be bought cheaply in the sports section of a supermarket. We have also provided a supplementary section of exercises which complement the main routines. The items of equipment required will all be found in a gym, but if you prefer to do the routines at home you will find that they can usually be performed on a simple, and relatively inexpensive, 'home gym'.

If you are worried about the cost of a home gym, you can look at the possibility of hiring one from a supplier of fitness equipment. Most of them hire out equipment at reasonable rates. Alternatively, check the price of a relatively cheap (but sturdy) home gym and compare it with the cost of a subscription to a commercial gymnasium: you may find that the investment in equipment is not so great after all!

However, don't worry if you are obliged to stick to the simple equipment mentioned here. You can get most of the benefit from the simpler exercises by following the instructions carefully, without having to outlay more than a few dollars. You can even improvise, if you wish. If you don't have a set of light dumbbells you can use a couple of short (say 20 cm or 8 in) lengths of metal pipe instead. As your proficiency improves, you may find the hollow pipe you are using as a barbell or dumbbells to be too light: in this case you can have someone fill the pipe (or fill it yourself if you're a handywoman) with cement or metal shot to make it heavier.

Similarly, if you don't have a bench for the flat-bench exercises, you can place a few sofa cushions on the floor and lay a folded ironing board on top of them to make an improvised bench. An incline bench can be made up by leaning a length of wood or pineboard—say 25 cm (10 in) by 60 cm (2 feet)—at an angle against the back of a chair. And so on. A little ingenuity will enable you to think up ways of creating your own 'home gym' without buying any special weight-training equipment at all.

I've heard it all before

Not another fitness craze! . . . We know what you're probably think-ing. This is just another of those 'crazes' or 'fads' that crop up regularly on TV or in monthly lifestyle or fitness magazines. Like some diets it's one of those fashions that come and go every few months, but never seem to stand the test of time!

We understand your scepticism, but we believe it isn't justified. To explain why, let us give you some facts about the exercise system you will find in this book. It is called the Matrix System.

ABOUT THE MATRIX SYSTEM

The Matrix System was invented and developed by Professor Ron Laura, Professor of Education at the University of Newcastle, New South Wales. A former champion weightlifter and experienced fitness instructor, he has been internationally recognised for his contributions in the field of weight training. The Matrix System, then, has been devised by one of the world's leading authorities in the field. The scientific principles on which it is based have been fully set out in our book *The Matrix Principle* (Allen & Unwin, 1991).

The system has been developed and refined over more than a decade in controlled tests at Harvard University, USA, and in fitness centres in Australia. The testing procedure involved hundreds of subjects, who were compared in trial programs to trainers using conventional weight methods. On average, five out of six subjects in the Matrix groups showed gains in strength and muscle growth significantly greater than in the conventional group, and the muscle gain of some Matrix trainers was three times that of conventional trainers. (A full description of the trials is given in the book mentioned above.)

The complete Matrix System consists of 36 exercise techniques (or

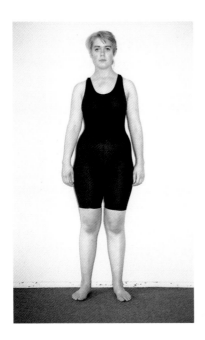 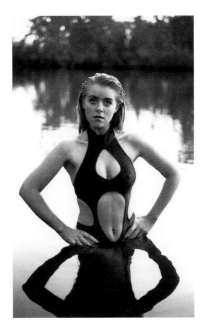

Julia Johnston before and after her twelve week Matrix program.

patterns of movement). Each technique represents an increasing level of difficulty, so the program of progressive resistance which it offers is systematic and safe. In this introductory twelve-week program we show how you can use the first twelve Matrix techniques to rejuvenate and reshape your body into one that you can be proud of.

IT HAS PROVED ITS EFFECTIVENESS

The Matrix System has been used by all kinds of trainers, men and women, from raw beginners to professional sportspeople and bodybuilders. It has been used by international sporting teams as part of their training regime, and we have shown how it can be applied to 25 different sports in our book *Weight Training for Sports* (Bantam, 1992).

The above background, we hope, will indicate that this is not a new exercise 'fad' without any credentials other than its novelty, but is a rigorously tested and proven *new approach* to resistance training which is gaining increasing recognition as more and more exercisers discover its effectiveness.

IT CAN'T REALLY BE THAT SIMPLE

In basic concept, it *is* simple. Matrix training takes the emphasis away from the use of heavy weights, and places it on the movement of the body—this movement being broken down into a number of component parts.

It's the *explanation* that is complex, and there isn't room in this practical manual to go into it in depth. For the interested reader, we have explained the physiological details in our earlier books—*The Matrix Principle* and *Matrix for Muscle Gain* (Allen & Unwin, 1993). Broadly speaking, the system has to do with the stopping and holding of movements at points where the muscles have to work hardest.

A GENUINE BREAKTHROUGH

In *practical* terms, however, it represents a real breakthrough, because it means that *you don't use heavy weights.* You can actually use extremely light weights, or in some cases your own body weight, to get the same effect as can only be achieved in conventional resistance training by the use of moderate-to-heavy weights.

This means that:

• it is suitable for women, children, older people and those who have never used weights before;
• the risk of strains and injuries is minimised;
• you can gradually build up the *intensity* of the exercise (without increasing the weights), thus increasing its cardiovascular benefit.

Add to all this the fact that it has been shown to work faster and more effectively than conventional resistance exercise, and you will see what a revolution Matrix training represents in the world of exercise.

A FEW MINUTES A DAY?

Maybe a little more than this, but most of us can spare a little of our time in the cause of health, fitness and a better looking body.

The preferred mode is to exercise for at least *fifteen to twenty* minutes *three* days each week. If you are pressed for time, you can split up your routine so that you do ten minutes in the morning and ten minutes in the afternoon or at night, as you wish. Since Matrix training takes so little time, hardly anyone can truthfully say 'I don't have enough time to do it'. The simple fact is that if you want to stay healthy and fit you have to exercise. Yes, it takes time, but Matrix training takes a quarter of the time and produces faster results than conventional training, so that it actually enables you to get the maximum benefit without *wasting* time.

You will need to take a few minutes to warm up before you begin the exercises, and the amount of time you take will obviously depend on how *intensively* you do them—that is, on how short a break you take between each exercise.

One of the distinguishing features of Matrix as compared to conventional weight exercise is that, by using high intensity rather than heavy weight to challenge the muscles into response, it avoids many of the problems associated with heavy weight, such as strains, tears and other injuries.

Moreover, by enabling the trainer to determine the intensity of the exercise, it puts the trainer more effectively in control of what is happening. You can use your body's 'feedback' to tell you whether you are working hard enough or whether (with the same weight) you could be adding to the challenge of the exercise you are doing. With conventional exercise, the only way of adding to the challenge is by adding more weight and thus increasing the risk of strain.

Intensity is an important part of Matrix exercise, and its effectiveness depends in large part on the very short pauses that you will see set out in the instructions.

GETTING USED TO IT

Don't worry if at first you need to pause a little longer than shown in the instructions. Your body is not used to Matrix exercise—it may not be used to serious exercise at all—and it will take a little time to become accustomed to the novel demands being made on it.

The body is remarkably adaptable, and learns quickly. It won't be long (provided you persevere) before you can cut down the breaks within and between exercises to the number of seconds specified. *This must be your primary goal*—it is far more important to reach the stage where you can do the exercise as set out (with the short pauses shown) than to increase the weight.

A HIGH-EFFICIENCY SYSTEM

Remember: weight is not the critical factor in Matrix exercise (though

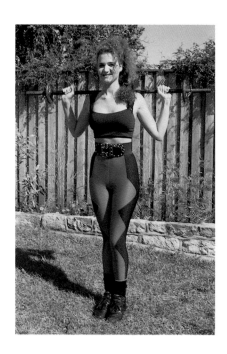

Sharon Laura takes advantage
of her back garden for a
morning training session.

you'll soon find your 'beginning' weight too light): what is critical is
the *pattern of movements* and the *short duration of the pauses*.

What this means is that, as your proficiency improves, you'll get
through your exercise session in increasingly shorter periods, because
your pauses will become briefer and briefer.

By the time you can do the exercises as specified you may even
wonder whether you're spending enough time on your exercise
session. In all probability you are—the clinical trials of the Matrix
System have shown that a 15 to 20 minute session (if done strictly)
can have a 'workout effect' equivalent to more than an hour of
conventional weight exercise.

So what can I expect?

A miraculous transformation in twelve weeks? . . We'd like to be able to say yes, but unfortunately it's just not the case. There are no 'miracles' in the world of exercise, just as there are no 'miracle cures' in the world of medicine.

Matrix exercise is certainly revolutionary and, we believe, more effective than any other resistance training method yet devised, but it works at the level of human physiology—not at that of the supernatural or the miraculous!

In fact, and at the risk of further disappointing you, you will probably notice no change at all in your appearance for the first four or even five weeks.

A 'BETTER BODY' WILL START TO EMERGE

This point is crucially important. Do not expect changes 'overnight': they don't happen. The body takes a few weeks to respond to the new demands being made upon it by altering its pattern of cellular adaptation: it has to 'realise', as it were, that these demands are not a *one-off stress* with which it can cope by a greater than usual effort, but that they have become part of the *regular pattern* of activity in which it is now engaged.

After a few weeks, the body begins to respond. It prepares itself for its regular 'dose' of exercise by becoming stronger and firmer. At first, you will notice these changes by *feeling* the new strength and firmness in the limbs, even if there's still quite a bit of flab covering the muscles underneath. Later you will begin to *see* the change as you look in the mirror, and you will even be able to apply the 'tape-measure test' to make sure that your eyes are not deceiving you.

WON'T I FEEL SORE?

At first, probably yes. Especially if you haven't exercised before, you may notice a certain soreness in the body parts you have been exercising.

You may feel a little tiredness, or even a mild pain, in the limbs as you do some exercises. This is perfectly normal, and is due to the build-up of lactic acid that occurs when we train with weights. It only lasts a few seconds, and if we pause for a short time most of the lactic acid is flushed away so that we can continue the exercise. You will notice this effect less and less as you grow accustomed to exercising, and soon you won't have to pause in the middle of what you're doing—you can do the exercise as instructed.

Not only will you feel less lactic acid pain as your fitness increases, you will at the same time be mobilising—and thus using up—more fat. In fact, the build-up of lactic acid in the blood causes a shift from fat to carbohydrate metabolism, once we reach what is called the 'lactate threshold'. At this point, lactate production exceeds removal and causes fat to be less available for muscle metabolism. One of the important effects of exercise is that you can do more and more of it (as your fitness improves) *before* lactic acid accumulates in the blood. The result of this is that more and more fat can be mobilised and used up: in other words, the fitter you are, the greater the percentage of your energy output that is derived from burning up fat. In fit exercisers, up to 90 per cent of the energy used is derived from fat rather than other sources—which is what we mean when we say that 'muscle burns fat'.

RESIDUAL SORENESS

The other kind of soreness occurs anything from 8 to 24 hours after exercise—a kind of 'tender soreness' in the limbs, which may last for a day or two. This also is perfectly normal: it's simply the sign that we are putting a new pattern of stress on the muscles.

This 'residual muscular soreness', as it is called, is not only different from the local discomfort that you may experience during exercise, it should also be differentiated from the acute pain which is a sign of muscle strain (a tear in the muscle fibre). If you do the exercises as instructed, sticking to light weights until your strength improves, you will minimise the risk of muscle strain. Should the latter occur, you should not try to 'work through it' but leave it to heal until the pain has disappeared.

Residual soreness tends to be associated with the 'negative' phase of exercise movements—that is, the phase in which a muscle is stretched rather than when it is contracted. In this negative phase the muscle fibres are exerting a more than usually heavy pull on connective tissue, causing the gradual development of mild local oedema (an increase in intercellular fluid) which is of no great concern and will pass off within a day or two.

Once again, residual soreness becomes less and less noticeable as we grow accustomed to exercise—though it may reappear after an extended layoff. Gently moving and/or massaging the area in question will usually provide relief.

WHAT IF I'M TEMPTED TO GIVE UP?

In one word: persevere. Take our word for it—it really does get easier as you go along. There is no hiding the fact that, if you are unfit when you start out, the first phase of your exercise regime will be marked by a certain amount of physical discomfort.

At this early stage, you will need to use every motivational trick you can. Whether it's that unflattering photo of yourself that you stick prominently to the door of the fridge, or the photo of someone who is the role model for how you'd like to look, you're probably the best judge of what motivational aid works best for you. It may help if you can exercise with a partner or friend who shares the same goals as you. Apart from the opportunity to motivate each other, the chances are that on days when you're tempted to drop out your partner will not be. You may even be the one who shames your training partner into not opting out of their regular exercise session.

Once you move on to phase two, the worst is over. As your body accustoms itself to exercise and your fitness improves, you'll begin to enjoy your workouts more. Not only will your level of discomfort drop, but you'll actually begin to enjoy that post-workout feeling of well-being—and even begin to notice the first visible results.

A recent survey by an Australian women's magazine reported that almost half (49 per cent) of exercising women regarded it primarily as a pleasure; the next largest group (37 per cent) saw it as an important discipline, and only 14 per cent thought of it as a necessary evil. Other surveys by behavioural scientists suggest that the more accustomed you become to exercise, the more you tend to pass from the third or second group into the first: you actually begin to look forward to your regular exercise session, even to get a 'high' from it.

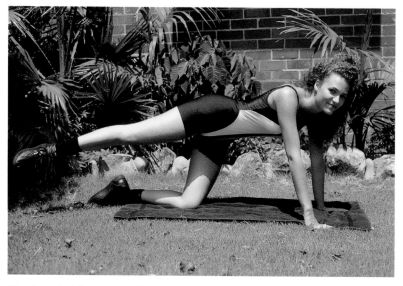

The leg stretch is a gentle warm-up exercise.

So, we repeat: don't give up. Stick with it through phase one, and the rest will take care of itself.

IS IT HARD TO FOLLOW?

It may at first *look* hard to follow, but you'll find it isn't once you grasp the principles of Matrix exercise. Look, for example, at the following diagram and assume that you are holding a light bar in your hands, which you are 'curling' up and down by bending your elbows.

Here is how the movement looks:

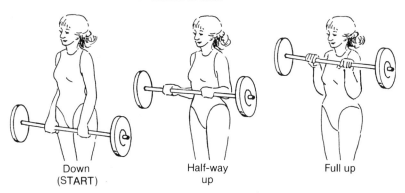

Down   Half-way   Full up
(START)   up

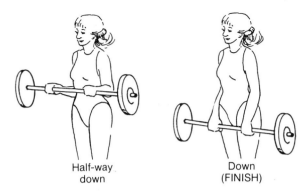

Half-way   Down
down   (FINISH)

Now for the pattern or sequence of movements (each movement is known as a 'rep' or repetition). Here is the sequence known as the 'Conventional' Matrix:

5 full reps
5 reps ½-up
5 reps ½-down
5 full reps

This means that you move the bar through its full range for 5 movements, then move it half-way up (and down again) for 5 movements, then bring it to the 'up' position and move it half-way down (and up again) for 5 movements, and finally move it through its full range for 5 movements.

We can represent this sequence in the following diagram:

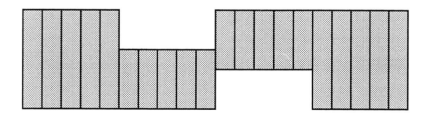

It may take some time to get used to the movement patterns, but don't be put off if at first they look difficult to follow. Each week has its own characteristic pattern of movements, and once you've done the first few exercises for the week (even if at first you have to keep referring to the text) you'll become familiar with that week's pattern and find it easy to remember. Each Matrix technique (or movement pattern) has its own underlying principle—such as an increasing number of reps or a decreasing number—and this will help you to memorise it readily.

Naturally, if you are training with a partner this will make things easier still: you can each do the exercises in turn, with the non-exercising partner reading out the instructions. Note, however, that you should perform the sequences as written, leaving only the short pauses specified (e.g. 30 or 40 seconds) between sets. So, if you are training with a partner, you will each need to do one complete body-part sequence (e.g. thighs and buttocks) in full before you and your partner switch roles.

WHAT IF I CAN'T KEEP UP?

Most exercisers will have no difficulty in following the program as set out. It has been extensively trialled with trainers in our Matrix clinics, many of them women who had never undertaken resistance training before. The overwhelming majority of them completed the twelve-week course on schedule with no problems.

A small number of trainers, however—particularly those who are unfit or very overweight—may find the progression from one week's pattern to the next week's (slightly more difficult) pattern a little too demanding. They should certainly not give up—after all, they are probably the ones most in need of an exercise regime—but rather readjust their sights and resolve to take a little longer to reach their goal. If you come into this category and find a particular weekly pattern beyond your capacity, just repeat the previous week's routines until your fitness level has improved further. (You can even go back to Week 1 if necessary.) Keep doing this, progressing at the rate you are comfortable with until you reach the goal. It is the *goal* that matters, even if it takes you a little longer to reach it. Remember that you will still be making progress, even if you stay with a particular weekly routine for a few weeks before moving on.

AND AFTER TWELVE WEEKS

As we've already said, you should start to feel an improvement in your general body tone before the end of this twelve-week course, and as you approach the end of it the difference should become visible. Not everyone makes progress at the same rate, however. Every body is different, and much will depend on how out-of-shape you

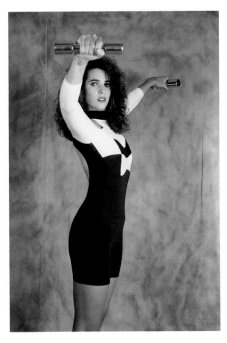

Helene Laura demonstrates the top position for the Side Lateral Raise, one of the movements used in the twelve week program.

were to begin with. Some exercisers will note a more rapid improvement than this, others less so. If you come into the latter category, *persevere*: the results will follow, even if a little more slowly in your case.

At the end of the twelve-week course we hope you'll feel inspired to maintain your exercise program. By now, your body will be used to its exercise routine and progress should continue. In our experience, it will be even more rapid from this point on.

To continue your exercise program beyond the twelfth week, we suggest that you return to the routines given for Week 9; the following week, move to Week 10, and so on. Weeks 9–12 will give you a self-contained four–week program which you can complete each month from now on. Each time you undertake the monthly program you should find that you can complete it more easily than last month. Don't rest on your laurels, however: increase the weights slightly, and/or increase the intensity by cutting down the pauses. Continue this program for as long as you like, and you'll maintain the trimmer, more active body you've been looking for.

Getting started

Do I need to warm up? . . . Yes, you do. It is never sensible to launch straight into your weight exercises, even if you are pressed for time. It increases the risk of muscle strain and injury, and prevents you from gaining the optimum benefit from your weight regime that comes from exercising with muscles that have been prepared for action.

It will only take a few minutes, perhaps as little as two or three in warm weather. The colder the weather, the longer you should spend in warming up. Unless the weather is hot it is a good idea to keep your body well covered for the warm-up—track pants and top are best. You can get down to your gymwear once you are fully into your workout and your body temperature has increased.

We suggest that your main warm-up activity should consist of either rope-jumping or jogging on the spot carried out at moderate pace for two to three minutes. If you don't have the co-ordination for rope jumping, or are not yet fit enough to jog on the spot for a few minutes, you can replace one of these activities by the body movements and stretching exercises listed below. The main thing is to loosen your joints and get the blood circulating more freely into the muscles.

Use these few minutes as an opportunity for mental relaxation as well. Forget about what you've just been doing or what you have to do later, and concentrate on becoming aware of your body. Feel the sheer sensual pleasure of the free movement of your limbs or even a good stretch.

Body movements
1   Stand with feet a short distance apart, hands on hips. Put your right foot out to one side and bring the left foot in. Then do the

same movement with the left foot leading. Perform this routine 10 times.

2 Walk on the spot for 20 counts, bring your knee well up at each stride.

3 Repeat 1.

4 Circle your shoulders backward 10 times.

5 Circle first one arm, then the other, backward. Do this 10 times, alternating arms.

6 With hands on hips and feet slightly apart, circle your hips to the right, backwards, to the left and forwards. Then rotate hips in the opposite direction. Do this 5 times, keeping the stomach tucked in as far as possible.

7 Standing with feet apart and toes slightly turned out, slowly bend your knees and lower your body as far as is comfortable, then straighten up. Repeat 10 times.

Stretching exercise

1 With feet slightly apart and hands on hips, step forward with one foot keeping the heel of the other foot on the ground. Bend the front knee to shift your weight forward. Hold for 10 seconds, then repeat with the other leg. Do this 3 times with each leg.

2 Stand upright, holding on to a chair or wall in front of you for support. In this posture, bring your right foot up towards your buttocks and clasp it with your hand. Hold for 10 seconds, feeling the muscle stretch in the front of your thigh. Repeat with the other leg. Do this 3 times with each leg.

3 Lie on your back with feet flat on the floor, knees bent. Raise one leg, clasp the back of the thigh and pull it towards your chest. Then stretch the leg towards the ceiling and hold for 10 seconds, feeling the muscle stretch in the back of your thigh. Repeat with the other leg. Do this 3 times with each leg.

THE EXERCISES

All the exercise movements used in the program are simple to perform and will become easier as you get used to them. They are all illustrated in the following pages, and a brief description of each is set out below:

1 *Floor Hyperextensions or Prone Lift of Legs*
Lie on the floor face-down, with your hands at the side of head, touching the floor. Keeping your upper body flat against the floor, raise your legs up as high as you can without feeling any pinching

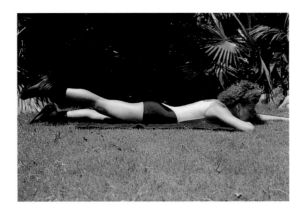

Prone Lift of the legs

sensation in your back. Don't overextend. Lower your legs and repeat the movement.

2 *Floor Hyperextensions or Prone Lift of Head*
As for prone lift of legs, but in this exercise the legs stay flat to the floor while you raise the trunk of your body, bending at the lower back. Again, don't overextend.

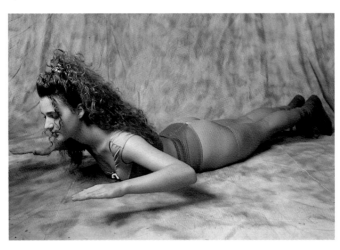

Prone Lift of the head

3 *Rear Squat*
Place a broomstick or length of pipe behind your neck. With feet shoulder-width apart and toes turned slightly out, bend the knees and lower the body till the thighs are parallel to the floor. Push up again, keeping the back straight and the head held up throughout the movement.

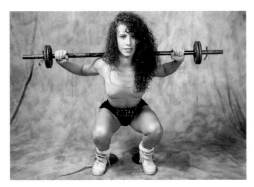

Rear Squat

4 Donkey Calf Raises

The exercise is so named because the trainer assumes a bent-over position which allows for a training partner to ride the back of the trainer in donkey fashion. The donkey calf raise illustrated assumes the donkey position but the rider is optional. Stand in a bent-over position, with your forearms on the back of a chair or other piece of furniture of appropriate height. Rest the balls of your feet on the edge of a solid block of wood or platform. Lower your heels as far as possible, then rise up on your toes as far as possible. Your knees should be slightly bent throughout the exercise. Stand with the toes pointing out for one set; then point them in for the next set.

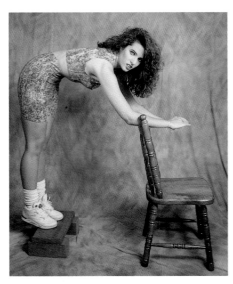

Donkey Calf Raises

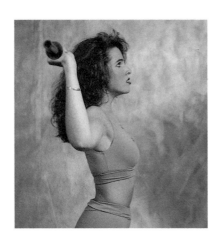

Roll Press Behind the Neck

5 *Roll Press Behind the Neck*

Place a broomstick or length of pipe behind your neck. With hands spaced slightly wider than shoulder-width apart, press the bar up in a single movement so that it travels above the head and down again onto the top of the chest. When viewed from the side, the movement should resemble an upside-down letter U. Return the bar in the same arc from the top of the chest to behind the neck. The movement from behind the shoulders to the chest and back again to the shoulder position makes up a single repetition.

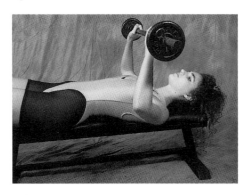

Bench Press

6 *Bench Press*

Lie face up on a flat bench, and position yourself so that your eyes are directly under the bar or length of pipe. Use a hand grip on the bar which is slightly wider than shoulder-width. Breathe in as you lower the bar or pipe to the chest and exhale on the way up.

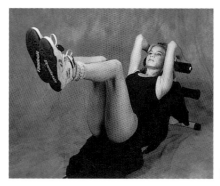

Incline Bench Leg Raise

7 *Incline Bench Leg Raise*

Lie on your back on an incline bench or board, with your head higher than your feet. Reach behind your head to grasp the top of the bench or board for support. Keeping your legs together and slightly bent at the knees, raise your legs towards your head to form a 90 degree angle. If you are able, lift your pelvis so that your bottom is lifted off the bench. From this position lower your legs slowly until they return to the starting position.

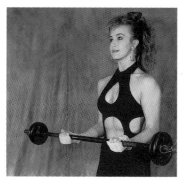
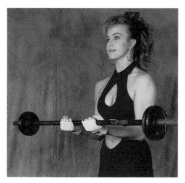

Wide Grip Biceps Curl (*left*) and Narrow Grip Biceps Curl (*right*)

8 *Wide Grip Biceps Curl*

Stand with feet slightly apart and grasp the bar or broomstick with hands about 40 cm (15 in) apart. Curl the bar up towards the shoulders, keeping the upper arm close in to the body and as stationary as possible. Try not to sway the body.

9 *Narrow Grip Biceps Curl*

As for wide grip biceps curl, but with hands holding the bar about 10 cm (4 in) apart.

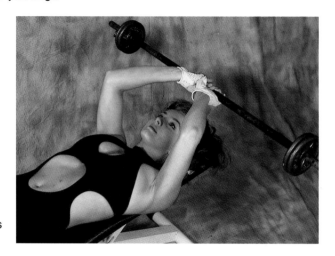

Narrow Grip
Lying Triceps
Press

10 *Narrow Grip Lying Triceps Press*
Lie on a bench, with knees bent and feet resting on the bench. Grasp
the bar or broomstick at arm's length with an overhand grip. Moving
the position of the upper arm as little as possible, bend your elbows
and slowly lower the bar towards the forehead, continuing till the bar
is slightly behind the head. Then return the bar to the starting position.

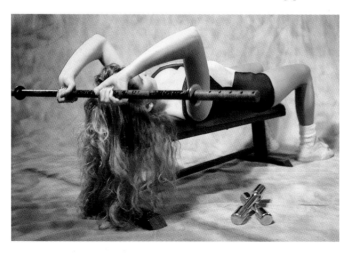

Medium
Grip
Lying
Triceps
Press

11 *Medium Grip Lying Triceps Press*
The same as for the narrow grip lying triceps press, but with hands
on the bar about 30 cm (12 in) apart.

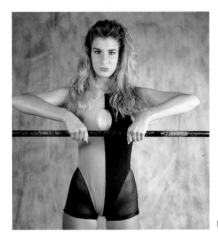

Upright Row

12 *Upright Row*
Stand holding the bar or stick in front of your thighs with an overhand grip, hands three finger-widths apart. Lift the bar until it almost touches your chin. Lower the bar again, keeping the body as still as possible and not swinging or throwing the weight up.

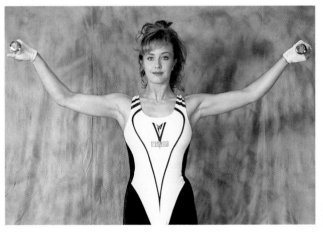

Lateral
Raise

13 *Lateral Raise*
Take a dumbbell in each hand, holding them together in front of your body. Raise the arms slowly to slightly above shoulder height, being careful not to swing the weights so as to use momentum. Lower the weights again slowly. Keep the elbows slightly unlocked throughout the movement.

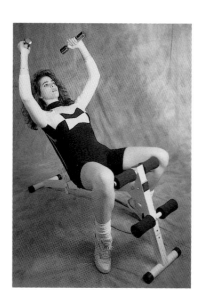

Incline Bench Press

14 *Incline Bench Press*
This is similar to the ordinary bench press, but is performed with your back resting against a bench or other support placed at a 45 degree angle. The bar or pipe is lifted from the chest and lowered again at an angle perpendicular to the floor. This exercise can also be done with dumbbells.

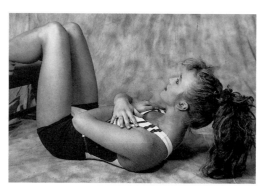

Abdominal Crunch

15 *Abdominal Crunch*
Lie on the floor with knees bent and anchored firmly against the wall. Alternatively, you can bend your knees and rest your lower legs on the seat of a chair. Place your hands on your chest—or behind your head (this makes the exercise harder)—and raise the head and shoul-

ders from the floor, curling the spine and contracting the abdominal muscles so as to crunch the upper and lower body together.

*   *   *

With the help of the above instructions and the illustrations, you should have no difficulty in performing the exercises listed below. The instructions for each exercise will show you how Matrix training works. And now it's time to see how it works for you. Make yourself a promise that next Monday will be the start of Week 1—the day you begin to take control of your body. Happy training!

Part II
The exercises

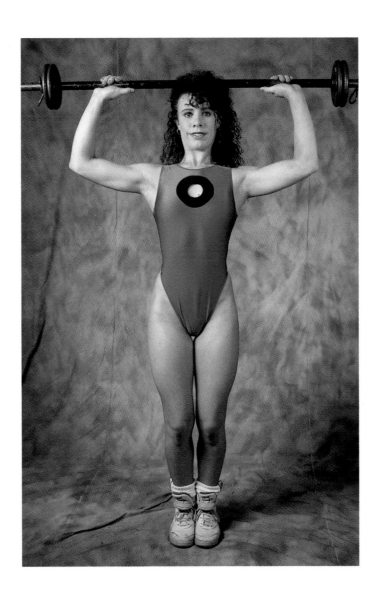

Week 1
The Conventional Matrix
Principle

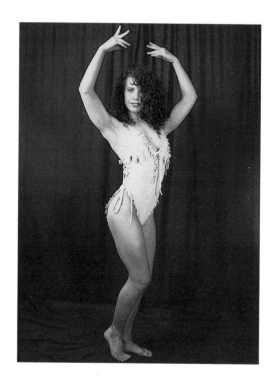

Tracey Moonen shows
the benefits of Matrix
training.

WEEK 1 – MONDAY

(Tick the box when you've completed the relevant exercise)

(a) Warm up options
Choose one type of warm up (see pages 34–35)   ☐

30 seconds pause

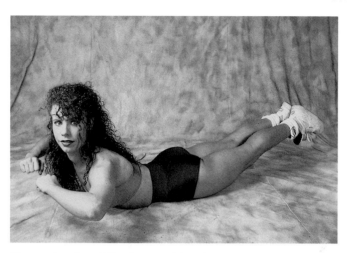

Hyperextension of the legs and head

(b) Lower back and buttocks training

1   *Conventional Matrix Floor Hyperextensions or Prone Lift of
    legs*
    5 full reps, 5 reps ½ up, 5 reps ½ down, 5 full reps   ☐

30 seconds pause

2   *Conventional Matrix Floor Hyperextensions or Prone Lift of
    head*
    5 full reps, 5 reps ½ up, 5 reps ½ down, 5 full reps   ☐

Rest one minute

(c) Thighs and buttocks training

1   *Conventional Matrix Rear Squats* (with or without weight)
    5 full reps, 5 reps ½ up, 5 reps ½ down, 5 full reps   ☐

40 seconds pause

2   *Conventional Matrix Rear Squats* (with or without weight)
    5 full reps, 5 reps ½ up, 5 reps ½ down, 5 full reps   ☐

Rest one minute

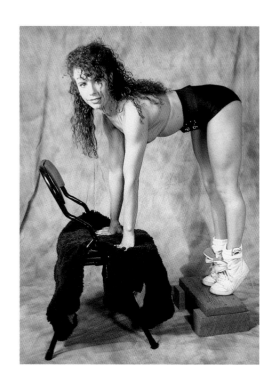

A Donkey Calf Raise in
the top position

(d) Calves training

1   *Conventional Matrix Donkey Calf Raises*
    5 full reps, 5 reps ½ up, 5 reps ½ down, 5 full reps   ☐

30 seconds pause

2   *Conventional Matrix Donkey Calf Raises*
    5 full reps, 5 reps ½ up, 5 reps down, 5 full reps   ☐

FINISH

WEEK 1 – WEDNESDAY

(Tick the box when you've completed the relevant exercise)

(a) Warm up options

(Choose one type of warm up, preferably different from the
previous day)   ☐

30 seconds pause

(b) Biceps training
1   *Conventional Matrix Wide Grip Biceps Curls*
     5 full reps, 5 reps ½ up, 5 reps ½ down, 5 full reps   ☐

20 seconds pause

2   *Conventional Matrix Narrow Grip Biceps Curls*
     5 full reps, 5 reps ½ up, 5 reps ½ down, 5 full reps   ☐

Rest one minute

(c) Triceps Training
1   *Conventional Matrix Narrow Grip Lying Triceps Press*
     5 full reps, 5 reps ½ up, 5 reps ½ down, 5 full reps   ☐

20 seconds pause

2   *Conventional Matrix Medium Grip Lying Triceps Press*
     5 full reps, 5 reps ½ up, 5 reps ½ down, 5 full reps,   ☐

FINISH

WEEK 1 – FRIDAY

(Tick the box when you've completed the relevant exercise)

(a) Warm up options
(Choose one type of warm up, preferably different from the
previous day)   ☐

30 seconds pause

(b) Shoulders, triceps and upper back training
1   *Conventional Matrix Upright Rows*
     5 full reps, 5 ½ up, 5 ½ down, 5 full reps   ☐

20 seconds pause

2   *Conventional Matrix Lateral Raises*
     5 full reps, 5 ½ up, 5 ½ down, 5 full reps   ☐

Rest one minute

(c) Chest, triceps and shoulders training

1   *Conventional Matrix Incline Bench Press*
    (Note: Can be done with dumbbells or a barbell)
    5 full reps, 5 reps ½ up, 5 reps ½ down, 5 full reps   ☐

20 seconds pause

2   *Conventional Matrix Incline Bench Press*
    5 full reps, 5 reps ½ up, 5 reps ½ down, 5 full reps   ☐

Rest one minute

(d) Midsection training

1   *Conventional Matrix Abdominal Crunch*
    5 full reps, 5 reps ½ up, 5 reps ½ down, 5 full reps   ☐

20 seconds pause

2   *Conventional Matrix Abdominal Crunch*
    5 full reps, 5 reps ½ up, 5 reps ½ down, 5 full reps   ☐

FINISH

Week 2
The Descending Matrix Principle

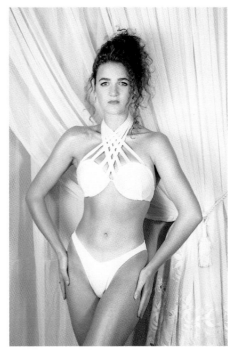

Sharon Laura has been using Matrix training for a number of years.

WEEK 2 – TUESDAY

(Tick the box when you've completed the relevant exercise)

(a) Warm up options
Choose one type of warm up (see pages 34–35) ☐

30 seconds pause

51

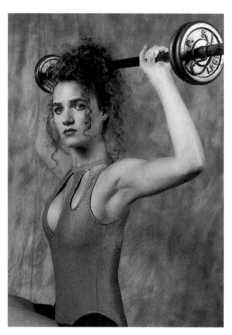

A Roll Press in the half-up position

(b) Shoulders, triceps and upper back training

1   *Descending Matrix Roll Press Behind the Neck*
    (Note: A broomstick or hollow length of pipe can be used)
    7 roll presses, 6 reps ½ up behind the neck, 5 reps ½
    down behind the neck, 4 roll presses   ☐

30 seconds pause

2   *Descending Matrix Roll Press Behind the Neck*
    7 roll presses, 6 reps ½ up behind the neck, 5 reps ½
    down behind the neck, 4 roll presses   ☐

Rest one minute

(c) Chest, triceps and shoulders training

1   *Descending Matrix Bench Press*
    7 full reps, 6 reps ½ up, 5 reps ½ down, 4 full reps   ☐

20 seconds pause

2   *Descending Matrix Bench Press*
    7 full reps, 6 reps ½ up, 5 reps ½ down, 4 full reps   ☐

Rest one minute

(d) Midsection training

1   *Descending Matrix Incline Bench Leg Raises*
    7 full reps, 6 reps ½ up, 5 reps ½ down, 4 full reps   ☐

20 seconds pause

2   *Descending Matrix Incline Bench Leg Raises*
    7 full reps, 6 reps ½ up, 5 reps ½ down, 4 full reps   ☐

FINISH

WEEK 2 – THURSDAY

(Tick the box when you've completed the relevant exercise)

(a) Warm up options
(Choose one type of warm up, preferably different from the
previous day)   ☐

30 seconds pause

(b) Lower back and buttocks training

1   *Descending Matrix Floor Hyperextensions or Prone Lift of
    legs*
    7 full reps, 6 reps ½ up, 5 reps ½ down, 4 full reps   ☐

30 seconds pause

2   *Descending Matrix Floor Hyperextensions or Prone Lift of
    head*
    7 full reps, 6 reps ½ up, 5 reps ½ down, 4 full reps   ☐

Rest one minute

(c) Thighs and buttocks training

1   *Descending Matrix Rear Squats*
    7 full reps, 6 reps ½ up, 5 reps ½ down, 4 full reps   ☐

40 seconds pause

2   *Descending Matrix Rear Squats*
    7 full reps, 6 reps ½ up, 5 reps ½ down, 4 full reps   ☐

Rest one minute

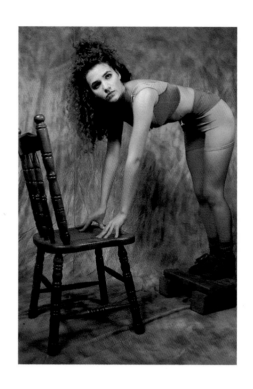

A Donkey Calf Raise in the
bottom position

(d) Calves training
1   *Descending Matrix Donkey Calf Raises*
    7 full reps, 6 reps ½ up, 5 reps ½ down, 4 full reps   ☐

30 seconds pause

2   *Descending Matrix Donkey Calf Raises*
    5 full reps, 5 reps ½ up, 5 reps ½ down, 5 full reps   ☐

FINISH

WEEK 2 – SATURDAY

(Tick the box when you've completed the relevant exercise)

(a) Warm up options
(Choose one type of warm up preferably different from the
previous day)   ☐

30 seconds pause

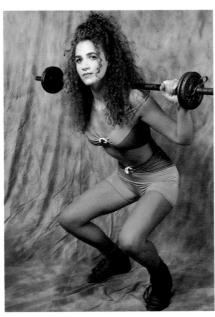

A Rear Squat in the half-up position

(b) Lower back and buttocks training

1   *Descending Matrix Floor Hyperextensions or Prone Lift of legs*
    7 full reps, 6 reps ½ up, 5 reps ½ down, 4 full reps   ☐

30 seconds pause

2   *Descending Matrix Floor Hyperextensions or Prone Lift of head*
    7 full reps, 6 reps ½ up, 5 up, 5 reps ½ down, 4 full reps   ☐

Rest one minute

(c) Thighs and buttocks training

1   *Descending Matrix Rear Squats* (with or without weight)
    7 full reps, 6 reps ½ up, 5 reps ½ down, 4 full reps   ☐

30 seconds pause

2   *Descending Matrix Rear Squats* (with or without weight)
    7 full reps, 6 reps ½ up, 5 reps ½ down, 4 full reps   ☐

Rest one minute

(d) Calves training

1   *Descending Matrix Donkey Calf Raises*
     7 full reps, 6 reps ½ up, 5 reps ½ down, 4 full reps   ☐

20 seconds pause

2   *Descending Matrix Donkey Calf Raises*
     7 full reps, 6 reps ½ up, 5 reps ½ down, 4 full reps   ☐

FINISH

Week 3
The Ascending Matrix
Principle

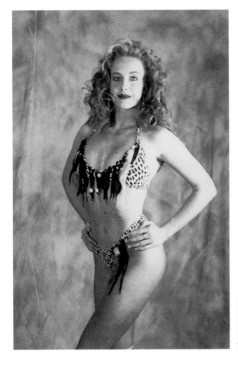

Sheridan Baldwin maintains a healthy lifestyle and undertakes regular Matrix training.

WEEK 3 – MONDAY

(Tick the box when you've completed the relevant exercise)

(a) Warm up options
Choose one type of warm up (see pages 34–35)   ☐

30 seconds pause

(b) Lower back and buttocks training

1   *Ascending Matrix Floor Hyperextensions or Prone Lift of legs*
    4 full reps, 5 reps ½ up, 6 reps ½ down, 7 full reps   ☐

30 seconds pause

2   *Ascending Matrix Floor Hyperextensions or Prone Lift of head*
    4 full reps, 5 reps ½ up, 6 reps ½ down, 7 full reps   ☐

Rest one minute

(c) Thighs and buttocks training

1   *Ascending Matrix Rear Squats* (with or without weight)
    4 full reps, 5 reps ½ up, 6 reps ½ down, 7 full reps   ☐

30 seconds pause

2   *Ascending Matrix Rear Squats* (with or without weight)
    4 full reps, 5 reps ½ up, 6 reps ½ down, 7 full reps   ☐

Rest one minute

(d) Calves training

1   *Ascending Matrix Donkey Calf Raises*
    4 full reps, 5 reps ½ up, 6 reps ½ down, 7 full reps   ☐

20 seconds pause

2   *Ascending Matrix Donkey Calf Raises*
    4 full reps, 5 reps ½ up, 6 reps ½ down, 7 full reps   ☐

FINISH

WEEK 3 – WEDNESDAY

(Tick the box when you've completed the relevant exercise)

(a) Warm up options
(Choose one type of warm up, preferably different from the previous day)   ☐

30 seconds pause

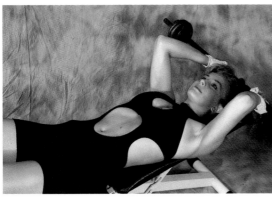

A Lying Triceps
Press in the
half-up position

(b) Biceps training

1   *Ascending Matrix Wide Grip Biceps Curls*
    4 full reps, 5 reps ½ up, 6 reps ½ down, 7 full reps   ☐

20 seconds pause

2   *Ascending Matrix Narrow Grip Biceps Curls*
    4 full reps, 5 reps ½ up, 6 reps ½ down, 7 full reps   ☐

Rest one minute

(c) Triceps training

1   *Ascending Matrix Narrow Grip Lying Triceps Press*
    4 full reps, 5 reps ½ up, 6 reps ½ down, 7 full reps   ☐

20 seconds pause

2   *Ascending Matrix Medium Grip Lying Triceps Press*
    4 full reps, 5 reps ½ up, 6 reps ½ down, 7 full reps   ☐

FINISH

WEEK 3 – FRIDAY

(Tick the box when you've completed the relevant exercise)

(a) Warm up options

(Choose one type of warm up, preferably different from the
previous day)   ☐

30 seconds pause

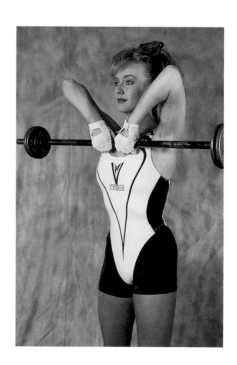

The top position of the Upright Row

(b) Shoulders, triceps and upper back training

1   *Ascending Matrix Upright Rows*
    4 full reps, 5 reps ½ up, 6 reps ½ down, 7 full reps   ☐

20 seconds pause

2   *Ascending Matrix Lateral Raises*
    4 full reps, 5 reps ½ up, 6 reps ½ down, 7 full reps   ☐

Rest one minute

(c) Chest, triceps and shoulders training

1   *Ascending Matrix Incline Bench Press*
    (Note: Can be done with dumbbells or a barbell)
    4 full reps, 5 reps ½ up, 6 reps ½ down, 7 full reps   ☐

20 seconds pause

2   *Ascending Matrix Incline Bench Press*
    4 full reps, 5 reps ½ up, 6 reps ½ down, 7 full reps   ☐

Rest one minute

(d) Midsection training

1   *Ascending Matrix Abdominal Crunch*
     4 full reps, 5 reps ½ up, 6 reps ½ down, 7 full reps   ☐

20 seconds pause

2   *Ascending Matrix Abdominal Crunch*
     4 full reps, 5 reps ½ up, 6 reps ½ down, 7 full reps   ☐

FINISH

Week 4
The Matrix Alternates
Principle

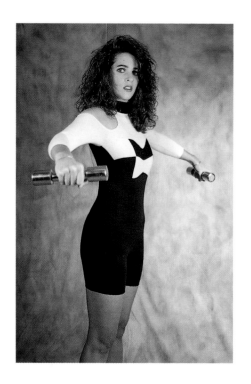

Helene Laura, demonstrating
Lateral Raises, finds time in
her busy life for regular
Matrix training.

WEEK 4 – TUESDAY

(Tick the box when you've completed the relevant exercise)

(a) Warm up options
Choose one type of warm up (see pages 34–35) ☐

30 seconds pause

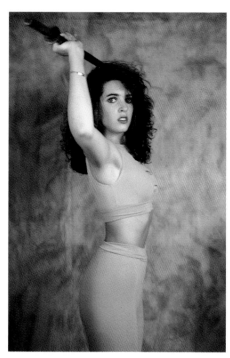

The top position in the Roll
Press movement

(b) Shoulders, triceps and upper back training

1 *Matrix Alternates Roll Press Behind the Neck*
   (Note: A broomstick or hollow length of pipe can be used)
5 roll presses   □
+

1 ½ up	1 ½ up	1 ½ up	1 ½ up	1 ½ up
1 ½ down +	1 ½ down +	1 ½ down +	1 ½ down	+ 1 ½ down
1 roll press	2 roll presses	3 roll presses	4 roll presses	5 roll presses

30 seconds pause

2 *Matrix Alternates Roll Press Behind the Neck*
5 roll presses   □
+

1 ½ up	1 ½ up	1 ½ up	1 ½ up	1 ½ up
1 ½ down +	1 ½ down +	1 ½ down +	1 ½ down	+ 1 ½ down
1 roll press	2 roll presses	3 roll presses	4 roll presses	5 roll presses

Rest one minute

(c) Chest, triceps and shoulders training

1   *Matrix Alternates Bench Press*
5 full reps   ☐
+

1 ½ up	1 ½ up	1 ½ up	1 ½ up	1 ½ up
1 ½ down +	1 ½ down +	1 ½ down +	1 ½ down +	1 ½ down
1 full rep	2 full reps	3 full reps	4 full reps	5 full reps

30 seconds pause

2   *Matrix Alternates Bench Press*
5 full reps   ☐
+

1 ½ up	1 ½ up	1 ½ up	1 ½ up	1 ½ up
1 ½ down +	1 ½ down +	1 ½ down +	1 ½ down +	1 ½ down
1 full rep	2 full reps	3 full reps	4 full reps	5 full reps

Rest one minute

(d) Midsection training

1   *Matrix Alternates Incline Bench Leg Raises*
5 full reps   ☐
+

1 ½ up	1 ½ up	1 ½ up	1 ½ up	1 ½ up
1 ½ down +	1 ½ down +	1 ½ down +	1 ½ down +	1 ½ down
1 full rep	2 full reps	3 full reps	4 full reps	5 full reps

20 seconds pause

2   *Matrix Alternates Incline Bench Leg Raises*
5 full reps   ☐
+

1 ½ up	1 ½ up	1 ½ up	1 ½ up	1 ½ up
1 ½ down +	1 ½ down +	1 ½ down +	1 ½ down +	1 ½ down
1 full rep	2 full reps	3 full reps	4 full reps	5 full reps

FINISH

WEEK 4 – THURSDAY

(Tick the box when you've completed the relevant exercise)

(a) Warm up options
(Choose one type of warm up, preferably different from the
previous day)   ☐

30 seconds pause

(b) Lower back and buttocks training
1   *Matrix Alternates Floor Hyperextensions or Prone Lift of legs*
5 full reps   ☐
+

1 ½ up	1 ½ up	1 ½ up	1 ½ up	1 ½ up
1 ½ down +	1 ½ down +	1 ½ down +	1 ½ down +	1 ½ down
1 full rep	2 full reps	3 full reps	4 full reps	5 full reps

30 seconds pause

2   *Matrix Alternates Floor Hyperextensions or Prone Lift of
    head*
5 full reps   ☐
+

1 ½ up	1 ½ up	1 ½ up	1 ½ up	1 ½ up
1 ½ down +	1 ½ down +	1 ½ down +	1 ½ down +	1 ½ down
1 full rep	2 full reps	3 full reps	4 full reps	5 full reps

Rest one minute

(c) Thighs and buttocks training
1   *Matrix Alternates Rear Squats*
5 full reps   ☐
+

1 ½ up	1 ½ up	1 ½ up	1 ½ up	1 ½ up
1 ½ down +	1 ½ down +	1 ½ down +	1 ½ down +	1 ½ down
1 full rep	2 full reps	3 full reps	4 full reps	5 full reps

40 seconds pause

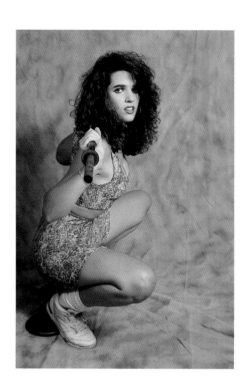

The bottom position for the
Rear Squat

2   *Matrix Alternates Rear Squats*
5 full reps   □
+

1 ½ up	1 ½ up	1 ½ up	1 ½ up	1 ½ up
1 ½ down +	1 ½ down +	1 ½ down +	1 ½ down +	1 ½ down
1 full rep	2 full reps	3 full reps	4 full reps	5 full reps

Rest one minute

(d) Calves training
1   *Matrix Alternates Donkey Calf Raises*
5 full reps   □
+

1 ½ up	1 ½ up	1 ½ up	1 ½ up	1 ½ up
1 ½ down +	1 ½ down +	1 ½ down +	1 ½ down +	1 ½ down
1 full rep	2 full reps	3 full reps	4 full reps	5 full reps

30 seconds pause

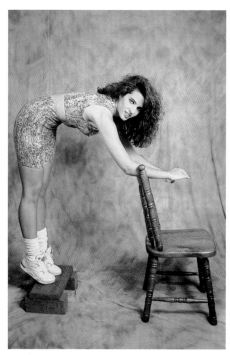

The Donkey Calf Raise
half-up

2   *Matrix Alternates Donkey Calf Raises*
5 full reps   ☐
+

1 ½ up	1 ½ up	1 ½ up	1 ½ up	1 ½ up
1 ½ down +	1 ½ down +	1 ½ down +	1 ½ down +	1 ½ down
1 full rep	2 full reps	3 full reps	4 full reps	5 full reps

FINISH

WEEK 4 – SATURDAY

(Tick the box when you've completed the relevant exercise)

(a) Warm up options
(Choose one type of warm up preferably different from the
previous day)   ☐

30 seconds pause

(b) Lower back and buttocks training

1   *Matrix Alternates Floor Hyperexensions or Prone Lift of legs*
5 full reps   ☐
+

1 ½ up	1 ½ up	1 ½ up	1 ½ up	1 ½ up
1 ½ down +	1 ½ down +	1 ½ down +	1 ½ down	+ 1 ½ down
1 full rep	2 full reps	3 full reps	4 full reps	5 full reps

30 seconds pause

2   *Matrix Alternates Floor Hyperexensions or Prone Lift of
      head*
5 full reps   ☐
+

1 ½ up	1 ½ up	1 ½ up	1 ½ up	1 ½ up
1 ½ down +	1 ½ down +	1 ½ down +	1 ½ down	+ 1 ½ down
1 full rep	2 full reps	3 full reps	4 full reps	5 full reps

Rest one minute

(c) Thighs and buttocks training

1   *Matrix Alternates Rear Squats* (with or without weight)
5 full reps   ☐
+

1 ½ up	1 ½ up	1 ½ up	1 ½ up	1 ½ up
1 ½ down +	1 ½ down +	1 ½ down +	1 ½ down	+ 1 ½ down
1 full rep	2 full reps	3 full reps	4 full reps	5 full reps

30 seconds pause

2   *Matrix Alternates Rear Squats* (with or without weight)
5 full reps   ☐
+

1 ½ up	1 ½ up	1 ½ up	1 ½ up	1 ½ up
1 ½ down +	1 ½ down +	1 ½ down +	1 ½ down	+ 1 ½ down
1 full rep	2 full reps	3 full reps	4 full reps	5 full reps

Rest one minute

(d) Calves training

1 *Matrix Alternates Donkey Calf Raises*

5 full reps   ☐

+

1 ½ up	1 ½ up	1 ½ up	1 ½ up	1 ½ up
1 ½ down +	1 ½ down +	1 ½ down +	1 ½ down +	1 ½ down
1 full rep	2 full reps	3 full reps	4 full reps	5 full reps

20 seconds pause

2 *Matrix Alternates Donkey Calf Raises*

5 full reps   ☐

+

1 ½ up	1 ½ up	1 ½ up	1 ½ up	1 ½ up
1 ½ down +	1 ½ down +	1 ½ down +	1 ½ down +	1 ½ down
1 full rep	2 full reps	3 full reps	4 full reps	5 full reps

FINISH

Week 5
The Cumulative Matrix
Principle

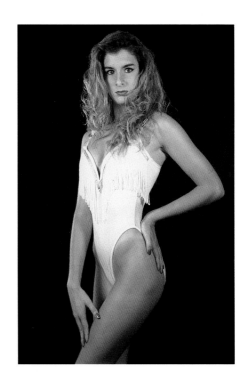

Melanie McGregor uses the
Matrix program to stay in
shape.

WEEK 5 – MONDAY

(Tick the box when you've completed the relevant exercise)

(a) Warm up options
Choose one type of warm up (see pages 34–35)　　　　　　☐

30 seconds pause

(b) Lower back and buttocks training

1   *Cumulative Matrix Floor Hyperextensions or Prone Lift of legs*

1 full rep	2 full reps	3 ½ up	4 ½ up
1 ½ up +	2 ½ up +	3 ½ down +	4 ½ down
1 ½ down	2 ½ down	4 full reps	5 full reps
	3 full reps		☐

30 seconds pause

2   *Cumulative Matrix Floor Hyperextensions or Prone Lift of head*

1 full rep	2 full reps	3 ½ up	4 ½ up
1 ½ up +	2 ½ up +	3 ½ down +	4 ½ down
1 ½ down	2 ½ down	4 full reps	5 full reps
	3 full reps		☐

Rest one minute

(c) Thighs and buttocks training

1   *Cumulative Matrix Rear Squats* (with or without weight)

1 full rep	2 full reps	3 ½ up	4 ½ up
1 ½ up +	2 ½ up +	3 ½ down +	4 ½ down
1 ½ down	2 ½ down	4 full reps	5 full reps
	3 full reps		☐

40 seconds pause

2   *Cumulative Matrix Rear Squats* (with or without weight)

1 full rep	2 full reps	3 ½ up	4 ½ up
1 ½ up +	2 ½ up +	3 ½ down +	4 ½ down
1 ½ down	2 ½ down	4 full reps	5 full reps
	3 full reps		☐

Rest one minute

(d) Calves training

1   *Cumulative Matrix Donkey Calf Raises*

1 full rep	2 full reps	3 ½ up	4 ½ up
1 ½ up +	2 ½ up +	3 ½ down +	4 ½ down
1 ½ down	2 ½ down	4 full reps	5 full reps
	3 full reps		☐

20 seconds pause

2   *Cumulative Matrix Donkey Calf Raises*

1 full rep	2 full reps	3 ½ up	4 ½ up
1 ½ up +	2 ½ up +	3 ½ down +	4 ½ down
1 ½ down	2 ½ down	4 full reps	5 full reps
	3 full reps		☐

FINISH

WEEK 5 – WEDNESDAY

(Tick the box when you've completed the relevant exercise)

(a) Warm up options
(Choose one type of warm up, preferably different from the
previous day)   ☐

30 seconds pause

(b) Biceps training
1   *Cumulative Matrix Wide Grip Biceps Curls*

1 full rep	2 full reps	3 ½ up	4 ½ up
1 ½ up +	2 ½ up +	3 ½ down +	4 ½ down
1 ½ down	2 ½ down	4 full reps	5 full reps
	3 full reps		☐

20 seconds pause

2   *Cumulative Matrix Narrow Grip Biceps Curls*

1 full rep	2 full reps	3 ½ up	4 ½ up
1 ½ up +	2 ½ up +	3 ½ down +	4 ½ down
1 ½ down	2 ½ down	4 full reps	5 full reps
	3 full reps		☐

Rest one minute

(c) Triceps training
1   *Cumulative Matrix Narrow Grip Lying Triceps Press*

1 full rep	2 full reps	3 ½ up	4 ½ up
1 ½ up +	2 ½ up +	3 ½ down +	4 ½ down
1 ½ down	2 ½ down	4 full reps	5 full reps
	3 full reps		☐

20 seconds pause

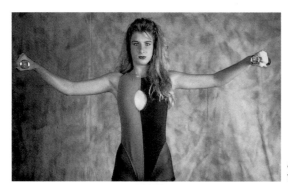

A Lateral Raise in
the half-up position

2   *Cumulative Matrix Medium Grip Lying Triceps Press*

1 full rep	2 full reps	3 ½ up	4 ½ up
1 ½ up +	2 ½ up +	3 ½ down +	4 ½ down
1 ½ down	2 ½ down	4 full reps	5 full reps
	3 full reps		☐

FINISH

WEEK 5 – FRIDAY

(Tick the box when you've completed the relevant exercise)

(a) Warm up options
(Choose one type of warm up, preferably different from the
previous day)   ☐

30 seconds pause

(b) Shoulders, triceps and upper back training
1   *Cumulative Matrix Upright Rows*

1 full rep	2 full reps	3 ½ up	4 ½ up
1 ½ up +	2 ½ up +	3 ½ down +	4 ½ down
1 ½ down	2 ½ down	4 full reps	5 full reps
	3 full reps		☐

20 seconds pause

2   *Cumulative Matrix Lateral Raises*

1 full rep	2 full reps	3 ½ up	4 ½ up
1 ½ up +	2 ½ up +	3 ½ down +	4 ½ down
1 ½ down	2 ½ down	4 full reps	5 full reps
	3 full reps		☐

Rest one minute

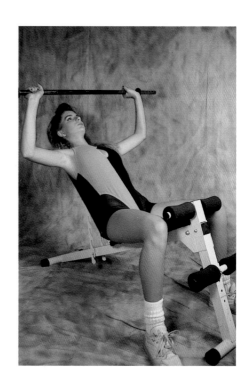

The Incline Bench Press in
the half-up position

(c) Chest, triceps and shoulders training

1   *Cumulative Matrix Incline Bench Press*
    (Note: Can be done with dumbbells or a barbell)

1 full rep	2 full reps	3 ½ up	4 ½ up
1 ½ up +	2 ½ up +	3 ½ down +	4 ½ down
1 ½ down	2 ½ down	4 full reps	5 full reps
	3 full reps		☐

20 seconds pause

2   *Cumulative Matrix Incline Bench Press*

1 full rep	2 full reps	3 ½ up	4 ½ up
1 ½ up +	2 ½ up +	3 ½ down +	4 ½ down
1 ½ down	2 ½ down	4 full reps	5 full reps
	3 full reps		☐

Rest one minute

(d) *Midsection training*

1   *Cumulative Matrix Abdominal Crunch*

1 full rep	2 full reps	3 ½ up	4 ½ up
1 ½ up +	2 ½ up +	3 ½ down +	4 ½ down
1 ½ down	2 ½ down	4 full reps	5 full reps
	3 full reps		☐

20 seconds pause

2   *Cumulative Matrix Abdominal Crunch*

1 full rep	2 full reps	3 ½ up	4 ½ up
1 ½ up +	2 ½ up +	3 ½ down +	4 ½ down
1 ½ down	2 ½ down	4 full reps	5 full reps
	3 full reps		☐

FINISH

Week 6
The Ladders Matrix
Principle

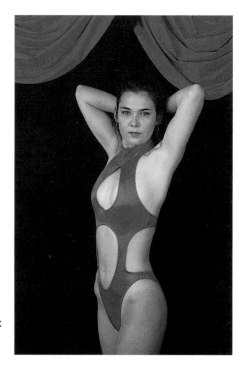

Jade Bennett uses the Matrix
program to stay fit and
healthy.

WEEK 6 – TUESDAY

(Tick the box when you've completed the relevant exercise)

(a) Warm up options
Choose one type of warm up (see pages 34–35)   ☐

30 seconds pause

(b) Shoulders, triceps and upper back training

1   *Ladders Matrix Roll Press Behind the Neck*
    (Note: A broomstick or hollow length of pipe can be used)

5 roll presses		1 rep ⅕ down
1 rep ⅕ up		1 rep ⅖ down
1 rep ⅖ up	+	1 rep ⅗ down
1 rep ⅗ up		1 rep ⅘ down
1 rep ⅘ up		1 roll press
1 roll press		5 roll presses ☐

30 seconds pause

2   *Ladders Matrix Roll Press Behind the Neck*

5 roll presses		1 rep ⅕ down
1 rep ⅕ up		1 rep ⅖ down
1 rep ⅖ up	+	1 rep ⅗ down
1 rep ⅗ up		1 rep ⅘ down
1 rep ⅘ up		1 roll press
1 roll press		5 roll presses ☐

Rest one minute

(c) Chest, triceps and shoulders training

1   *Ladders Matrix Bench Press*

5 full reps		1 rep ⅕ down
1 rep ⅕ up		1 rep ⅖ down
1 rep ⅖ up	+	1 rep ⅗ down
1 rep ⅗ up		1 rep ⅘ down
1 rep ⅘ up		1 full rep
1 full rep		5 full reps ☐

20 seconds pause

2   *Ladders Matrix Bench Press*

5 full reps		1 rep ⅕ down
1 rep ⅕ up		1 rep ⅖ down
1 rep ⅖ up	+	1 rep ⅗ down
1 rep ⅗ up		1 rep ⅘ down
1 rep ⅘ up		1 full rep
1 full rep		5 full reps ☐

Rest one minute

(d) Midsection training

1   Ladders Matrix Incline Bench Leg Raises

5 full reps	1 rep ⅕ down
1 rep ⅕ up	1 rep ⅖ down
1 rep ⅖ up +	1 rep ⅗ down
1 rep ⅗ up	1 rep ⅘ down
1 rep ⅘ up	1 full rep
1 full rep	5 full reps □

20 seconds pause

2   Ladders Matrix Incline Bench Leg Raises

5 full reps	1 rep ⅕ down
1 rep ⅕ up	1 rep ⅖ down
1 rep ⅖ up +	1 rep ⅗ down
1 rep ⅗ up	1 rep ⅘ down
1 rep ⅘ up	1 full rep
1 full rep	5 full reps □

FINISH

WEEK 6 – THURSDAY

(Tick the box when you've completed the relevant exercise)

(a) Warm up options
(Choose one type of warm up, preferably different from the previous day)   □

30 seconds pause

(b) Lower back and buttocks training

1   Ladders Matrix Floor Hyperextensions or Prone Lift of legs

5 full reps	1 rep ⅕ down
1 rep ⅕ up	1 rep ⅖ down
1 rep ⅖ up +	1 rep ⅗ down
1 rep ⅗ up	1 rep ⅘ down
1 rep ⅘ up	1 full rep
1 full rep	5 full reps □

30 seconds pause

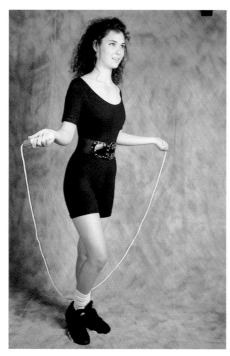

Warming up with a jump rope

2   *Ladders Matrix Floor Hyperextensions or Prone Lift of head*

5 full reps	1 rep ⅕ down
1 rep ⅕ up	1 rep ⅖ down
1 rep ⅖ up +	1 rep ⅗ down
1 rep ⅗ up	1 rep ⅘ down
1 rep ⅘ up	1 full rep
1 full rep	5 full reps ☐

Rest one minute

(c) Thighs and buttocks training

1   *Ladders Matrix Rear Squats*

5 full reps	1 rep ⅕ down
1 rep ⅕ up	1 rep ⅖ down
1 rep ⅖ up +	1 rep ⅗ down
1 rep ⅗ up	1 rep ⅘ down
1 rep ⅘ up	1 full rep
1 full rep	5 full reps ☐

40 seconds pause

2 *Ladders Matrix Rear Squats*

5 full reps		1 rep ⅕ down
1 rep ⅕ up		1 rep ⅖ down
1 rep ⅖ up	+	1 rep ⅗ down
1 rep ⅗ up		1 rep ⅘ down
1 rep ⅘ up		1 full rep
1 full rep		5 full reps	☐

Rest one minute

(d) Calves Training

1 *Ladders Matrix Donkey Calf Raises*

5 full reps		1 rep ⅕ down
1 rep ⅕ up		1 rep ⅖ down
1 rep ⅖ up	+	1 rep ⅗ down
1 rep ⅗ up		1 rep ⅘ down
1 rep ⅘ up		1 full rep
1 full rep		5 full reps	☐

30 seconds pause

2 *Ladders Matrix Donkey Calf Raises*

5 full reps		1 rep ⅕ down
1 rep ⅕ up		1 rep ⅖ down
1 rep ⅖ up	+	1 rep ⅗ down
1 rep ⅗ up		1 rep ⅘ down
1 rep ⅘ up		1 full rep
1 full rep		5 full reps	☐

FINISH

WEEK 6 – SATURDAY

(Tick the box when you've completed the relevant exercise)

(a) Warm up options

(Choose one type of warm up preferably different from the
previous day) ☐

30 seconds pause

(b) Lower back and buttocks training

1 *Ladders Matrix Floor Hyperextensions or Prone Lift of legs*

5 full reps		1 rep ⅕ down
1 rep ⅕ up		1 rep ⅖ down
1 rep ⅖ up	+	1 rep ⅗ down
1 rep ⅗ up		1 rep ⅘ down
1 rep ⅘ up		1 full rep
1 full rep		5 full reps □

30 seconds pause

2 *Ladders Matrix Floor Hyperextensions or Prone Lift of head*

5 full reps		1 rep ⅕ down
1 rep ⅕ up		1 rep ⅖ down
1 rep ⅖ up	+	1 rep ⅗ down
1 rep ⅗ up		1 rep ⅘ down
1 rep ⅘ up		1 full rep
1 full rep		5 full reps □

Rest one minute

(c) Thighs and buttocks training

1 *Ladders Matrix Rear Squats* (with or without weight)

5 full reps		1 rep ⅕ down
1 rep ⅕ up		1 rep ⅖ down
1 rep ⅖ up	+	1 rep ⅗ down
1 rep ⅗ up		1 rep ⅘ down
1 rep ⅘ up		1 full rep
1 full rep		5 full reps □

30 seconds pause

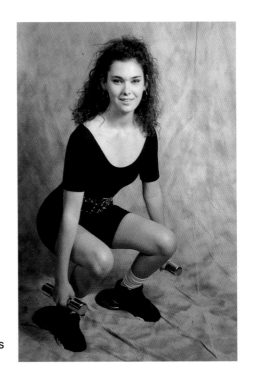

A Rear Squat with dumbbells
in the half-down position

2 *Ladders Matrix Rear Squats* (with or without weight)

5 full reps	1 rep ⅕ down
1 rep ⅕ up	1 rep ⅖ down
1 rep ⅖ up +	1 rep ⅗ down
1 rep ⅗ up	1 rep ⅘ down
1 rep ⅘ up	1 full rep
1 full rep	5 full reps □

Rest one minute

(d) Calves training

1 *Ladders Matrix Donkey Calf Raises*

5 full reps	1 rep ⅕ down
1 rep ⅕ up	1 rep ⅖ down
1 rep ⅖ up +	1 rep ⅗ down
1 rep ⅗ up	1 rep ⅘ down
1 rep ⅘ up	1 full rep
1 full rep	5 full reps □

20 seconds pause

2 *Ladders Matrix Donkey Calf Raises*

5 full reps		1 rep ⅕ down
1 rep ⅕ up		1 rep ⅖ down
1 rep ⅖ up	+	1 rep ⅗ down
1 rep ⅗ up		1 rep ⅘ down
1 rep ⅘ up		1 full rep
1 full rep		5 full reps

☐

FINISH

Week 7
The Cumulative Matrix
Ladders Principle

WEEK 7 – MONDAY

(Tick the box when you've completed the relevant exercise)

(a) Warm up options
Choose one type of warm up (see pages 34–35)   ☐

30 seconds pause

(b) Lower back and buttocks training
1 *Cumulative Matrix Ladders Floor Hyperextensions or Prone*
   Lift of legs

1 full rep	1 rep ⅕ down
1 rep ⅕ up	2 reps ⅖ down
2 reps ⅖ up +	3 reps ⅗ down
3 reps ⅗ up	4 reps ⅘ down
4 reps ⅘ up	5 full reps
5 full reps	

☐

30 seconds pause

2 *Cumulative Matrix Ladders Floor Hyperextensions or Prone*
   Lift of head

1 full rep	1 rep ⅕ down
1 rep ⅕ up	2 reps ⅖ down
2 reps ⅖ up +	3 reps ⅗ down
3 reps ⅗ up	4 reps ⅘ down
4 reps ⅘ up	5 full reps
5 full reps	

☐

Rest one minute

(c) Thighs and buttocks training

1 *Cumulative Matrix Ladders Rear Squats* (with or without weight)

1 full rep		1 rep ⅕ down
1 rep ⅕ up		2 reps ⅖ down
2 reps ⅖ up	+	3 reps ⅗ down
3 reps ⅗ up		4 reps ⅘ down
4 reps ⅘ up		5 full reps
5 full reps		

☐

40 seconds pause

2 *Cumulative Matrix Ladders Rear Squats* (with or without weight)

1 full rep		1 rep ⅕ down
1 rep ⅕ up		2 reps ⅖ down
2 reps ⅖ up	+	3 reps ⅗ down
3 reps ⅗ up		4 reps ⅘ down
4 reps ⅘ up		5 full reps
5 full reps		

☐

Rest one minute

(d) Calves training

1 *Cumulative Matrix Ladders Donkey Calf Raises*

1 full rep		1 rep ⅕ down
1 rep ⅕ up		2 reps ⅖ down
2 reps ⅖ up	+	3 reps ⅗ down
3 reps ⅗ up		4 reps ⅘ down
4 reps ⅘ up		5 full reps
5 full reps		

☐

20 seconds pause

2 *Cumulative Matrix Ladders Donkey Calf Raises*

1 full rep		1 rep ⅕ down
1 rep ⅕ up		2 reps ⅖ down
2 reps ⅖ up	+	3 reps ⅗ down
3 reps ⅗ up		4 reps ⅘ down
4 reps ⅘ up		5 full reps
5 full reps		

☐

FINISH

WEEK 7 – WEDNESDAY

(Tick the box when you've completed the relevant exercise)

(a) Warm up options
(Choose one type of warm up, preferably different from the previous day)   ☐

30 seconds pause

(b) Biceps training
1   *Cumulative Matrix Ladders Wide Grip Biceps Curls*

1 full rep	1 rep 1/5 down
1 rep 1/5 up	2 reps 2/5 down
2 reps 2/5 up +	3 reps 3/5 down
3 reps 3/5 up	4 reps 4/5 down
4 reps 4/5 up	5 full reps
5 full reps	☐

20 seconds pause

2   *Cumulative Matrix Ladders Narrow Grip Biceps Curls*

1 full rep	1 rep 1/5 down
1 rep 1/5 up	2 reps 2/5 down
2 reps 2/5 up +	3 reps 3/5 down
3 reps 3/5 up	4 reps 4/5 down
4 reps 4/5 up	5 full reps
5 full reps	☐

Rest one minute

(c) Triceps training
1   *Cumulative Matrix Ladders Narrow Grip Lying Triceps Press*

1 full rep	1 rep 1/5 down
1 rep 1/5 up	2 reps 2/5 down
2 reps 2/5 up +	3 reps 3/5 down
3 reps 3/5 up	4 reps 4/5 down
4 reps 4/5 up	5 full reps
5 full reps	☐

20 seconds pause

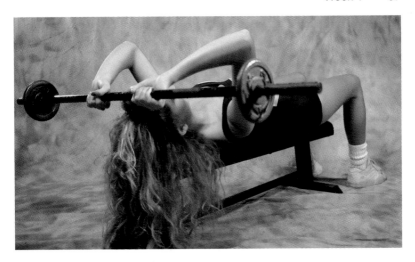

A Lying Triceps Press half-down

2   *Cumulative Matrix Ladders Medium Grip Lying Triceps Press*
　　1 full rep　　　　　　1 rep 1/5 down
　　1 rep 1/5 up　　　　　2 reps 2/5 down
　　2 reps 2/5 up　　+　　3 reps 3/5 down
　　3 reps 3/5 up　　　　　4 reps 4/5 down
　　4 reps 4/5 up　　　　　5 full reps
　　5 full reps　　　　　　　　　　　　□

FINISH

WEEK 7 – FRIDAY

(Tick the box when you've completed the relevant exercise)

(a) Warm up options
(Choose one type of warm up, preferably different from the
previous day)　　　　　　　　　　　　　　　□

30 seconds pause

(b) Shoulders, triceps and upper back training

1   *Cumulative Matrix Ladders Upright Rows*

1 full rep		1 rep ⅕ down
1 rep ⅕ up		2 reps ⅖ down
2 reps ⅖ up	+	3 reps ⅗ down
3 reps ⅗ up		4 reps ⅘ down
4 reps ⅘ up		5 full reps
5 full reps		

☐

20 seconds pause

2   *Cumulative Matrix Ladders Lateral Raises*

1 full rep		1 rep ⅕ down
1 rep ⅕ up		2 reps ⅖ down
2 reps ⅖ up	+	3 reps ⅗ down
3 reps ⅗ up		4 reps ⅘ down
4 reps ⅘ up		5 full reps
5 full reps		

☐

Rest one minute

(c) Chest, triceps and shoulders training

1   *Cumulative Matrix Ladders Incline Bench Press*
    (Note: Can be done with dumbbells or a barbell)

1 full rep		1 rep ⅕ down
1 rep ⅕ up		2 reps ⅖ down
2 reps ⅖ up	+	3 reps ⅗ down
3 reps ⅗ up		4 reps ⅘ down
4 reps ⅘ up		5 full reps
5 full reps		

☐

20 second pause

2   *Cumulative Matrix Ladders Incline Bench Press*

1 full rep		1 rep ⅕ down
1 rep ⅕ up		2 reps ⅖ down
2 reps ⅖ up	+	3 reps ⅗ down
3 reps ⅗ up		4 reps ⅘ down
4 reps ⅘ up		5 full reps
5 full reps		

☐

Rest one minute

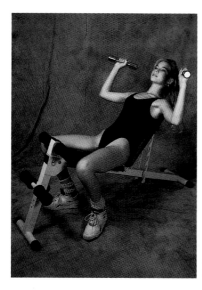

An Incline Bench Press with
dumbbells in the half-down position

(d) Midsection training

1   *Cumulative Matrix Ladders Abdominal Crunch*

1 full rep		1 rep ⅕ down
1 rep ⅕ up		2 reps ⅖ down
2 reps ⅖ up	+	3 reps ⅗ down
3 reps ⅗ up		4 reps ⅘ down
4 reps ⅘ up		5 full reps
5 full reps		☐

20 seconds pause

2   *Cumulative Matrix Ladders Abdominal Crunch*

1 full rep		1 rep ⅕ down
1 rep ⅕ up		2 reps ⅖ down
2 reps ⅖ up	+	3 reps ⅗ down
3 reps ⅗ up		4 reps ⅘ down
4 reps ⅘ up		5 full reps
5 full reps		☐

FINISH

Week 8
The Ascending
Iso-Matrix Principle

WEEK 8 – TUESDAY

(Tick the box when you've completed the relevant exercise)

(a) *Warm up options*
Choose one type of warm up (see pages 34–35)   ☐

30 seconds pause

(b) *Shoulders, triceps and upper back training*
1   *Ascending Iso-Matrix Roll Press Behind the Neck*
    (Note: A broomstick or hollow length of pipe can be used)
    5 roll presses
    1 rep ½ up (holding weight in the half position for 1 second)
    1 rep ½ up (hold for 2 seconds)
    1 rep ½ up (hold for 3 seconds)
    1 rep ½ up (hold for 4 seconds)
    1 rep ½ up (hold for 5 seconds)
    1 roll press
    +
    1 rep ½ down (holding weight in the half position for 1
    second)
    1 rep ½ down (hold for 2 seconds)
    1 rep ½ down (hold for 3 seconds)
    1 rep ½ down (hold for 4 seconds)
    1 rep ½ down (hold for 5 seconds)
    5 roll presses   ☐

30 seconds pause

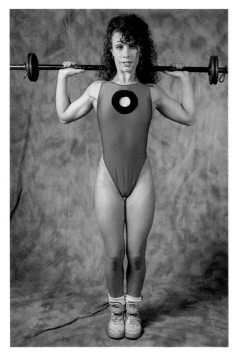

The starting position of the
Roll Press Behind the Neck

2   *Ascending Iso-Matrix Roll Press Behind the Neck*
    5 roll presses
    1 rep ½ up (holding weight in the half position for 1 second)
    1 rep ½ up (hold for 2 seconds)
    1 rep ½ up (hold for 3 seconds)
    1 rep ½ up (hold for 4 seconds)
    1 rep ½ up (hold for 5 seconds)
    1 roll press
    +
    1 rep ½ down (holding weight in the half position for 1
    second)
    1 rep ½ down (hold for 2 seconds)
    1 rep ½ down (hold for 3 seconds)
    1 rep ½ down (hold for 4 seconds)
    1 rep ½ down (hold for 5 seconds)
    5 roll presses   ☐

Rest one minute

(c) Chest, triceps and shoulders training

1   *Ascending Iso-Matrix Bench Press*
    5 full reps
    1 rep ½ up (holding weight in the half position for 1 second)
    1 rep ½ up (hold for 2 seconds)
    1 rep ½ up (hold for 3 seconds)
    1 rep ½ up (hold for 4 seconds)
    1 rep ½ up (hold for 5 seconds)
    1 full rep
    +
    1 rep ½ down (holding weight in the half position for 1 second)
    1 rep ½ down (hold for 2 seconds)
    1 rep ½ down (hold for 3 seconds)
    1 rep ½ down (hold for 4 seconds)
    1 rep ½ down (hold for 5 seconds)
    5 full reps   ☐

20 seconds pause

2   *Ascending Iso-Matrix Bench Press*
    5 full reps
    1 rep ½ up (holding weight in the half position for 1 second)
    1 rep ½ up (hold for 2 seconds)
    1 rep ½ up (hold for 3 seconds)
    1 rep ½ up (hold for 4 seconds)
    1 rep ½ up (hold for 5 seconds)
    1 full rep
    +
    1 rep ½ down (holding weight in the half position for 1 second)
    1 rep ½ down (hold for 2 seconds)
    1 rep ½ down (hold for 3 seconds)
    1 rep ½ down (hold for 4 seconds)
    1 rep ½ down (hold for 5 seconds)
    5 full reps   ☐

Rest one minute

(d) Midsection training

1 *Ascending Iso-Matrix Incline Bench Leg Raises*
   5 full reps
   1 rep ½ up (holding weight in the half position for 1 second)
   1 rep ½ up (hold for 2 seconds)
   1 rep ½ up (hold for 3 seconds)
   1 rep ½ up (hold for 4 seconds)
   1 rep ½ up (hold for 5 seconds)
   1 full rep
   +
   1 rep ½ down (holding weight in the half position for 1 second)
   1 rep ½ down (hold for 2 seconds)
   1 rep ½ down (hold for 3 seconds)
   1 rep ½ down (hold for 4 seconds)
   1 rep ½ down (hold for 5 seconds)
   5 full reps   □

20 seconds pause

2 *Ascending Iso-Matrix Incline Bench Leg Raises*
   5 full reps
   1 rep ½ up (holding weight in the half position for 1 second)
   1 rep ½ up (hold for 2 seconds)
   1 rep ½ up (hold for 3 seconds)
   1 rep ½ up (hold for 4 seconds)
   1 rep ½ up (hold for 5 seconds)
   1 full rep
   +
   1 rep ½ down (holding weight in the half position for 1 second)
   1 rep ½ down (hold for 2 seconds)
   1 rep ½ down (hold for 3 seconds)
   1 rep ½ down (hold for 4 seconds)
   1 rep ½ down (hold for 5 seconds)
   5 full reps   □

FINISH

WEEK 8 – THURSDAY

(Tick the box when you've completed the relevant exercise)

(a) Warm up options
(Choose one type of warm up, preferably different from the previous day).   ☐

30 seconds pause

(b) Lower back and buttocks training
1   *Ascending Iso-Matrix Floor Hyperextensions or Prone Lift of legs*
    5 full reps
    1 rep ½ up (holding weight in the half position for 1 second)
    1 rep ½ up (hold for 2 seconds)
    1 rep ½ up (hold for 3 seconds)
    1 rep ½ up (hold for 4 seconds)
    1 rep ½ up (hold for 5 seconds)
    1 full rep
    +
    1 rep ½ down (holding weight in the half position for 1 second)
    1 rep ½ down (hold for 2 seconds)
    1 rep ½ down (hold for 3 seconds)
    1 rep ½ down (hold for 4 seconds)
    1 rep ½ down (hold for 5 seconds)
    5 full reps   ☐

30 seconds pause

2   *Ascending Iso-Matrix Floor Hyperextensions or Prone Lift of head*
     5 full reps
     1 rep ½ up (holding weight in the half position for 1 second)
     1 rep ½ up (hold for 2 seconds)
     1 rep ½ up (hold for 3 seconds)
     1 rep ½ up (hold for 4 seconds)
     1 rep ½ up (hold for 5 seconds)
     1 full rep
     +
     1 rep ½ down (holding weight in the half position for 1 second)
     1 rep ½ down (hold for 2 seconds)
     1 rep ½ down (hold for 3 seconds)
     1 rep ½ down (hold for 4 seconds)
     1 rep ½ down (hold for 5 seconds)
     5 full reps   ☐

Rest one minute

(c) Thighs and buttocks training

1   *Ascending Iso-Matrix Rear Squats*
     5 full reps
     1 rep ½ up (holding weight in the half position for 1 second)
     1 rep ½ up (hold for 2 seconds)
     1 rep ½ up (hold for 3 seconds)
     1 rep ½ up (hold for 4 seconds)
     1 rep ½ up (hold for 5 seconds)
     1 full rep
     +
     1 rep ½ down (holding weight in the half position for 1 second)
     1 rep ½ down (hold for 2 seconds)
     1 rep ½ down (hold for 3 seconds)
     1 rep ½ down (hold for 4 seconds)
     1 rep ½ down (hold for 5 seconds)
     5 full reps   ☐

30 seconds pause

2   *Ascending Iso-Matrix Rear Squats*
     5 full reps
     1 rep ½ up (holding weight in the half position for 1 second)
     1 rep ½ up (hold for 2 seconds)
     1 rep ½ up (hold for 3 seconds)
     1 rep ½ up (hold for 4 seconds)
     1 rep ½ up (hold for 5 seconds)
     1 full rep
     +
     1 rep ½ down (holding weight in the half position for 1 second)
     1 rep ½ down (hold for 2 seconds)
     1 rep ½ down (hold for 3 seconds)
     1 rep ½ down (hold for 4 seconds)
     1 rep ½ down (hold for 5 seconds)
     5 full reps   □

Rest one minute

(d) Calves training
1   *Ascending Iso-Matrix Donkey Calf Raises*
     5 full reps
     1 rep ½ up (holding weight in the half position for 1 second)
     1 rep ½ up (hold for 2 seconds)
     1 rep ½ up (hold for 3 seconds)
     1 rep ½ up (hold for 4 seconds)
     1 rep ½ up (hold for 5 seconds)
     1 full rep
     +
     1 rep ½ down (holding weight in the half position for 1 second)
     1 rep ½ down (hold for 2 seconds)
     1 rep ½ down (hold for 3 seconds)
     1 rep ½ down (hold for 4 seconds)
     1 rep ½ down (hold for 5 seconds)
     5 full reps   □

30 seconds pause

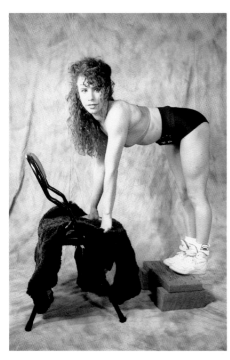

A Donkey Calf Raise in the bottom position

2   *Ascending Iso-Matrix Donkey Calf Raises*
5 full reps
1 rep ½ up (holding weight in the half position for 1 second)
1 rep ½ up (hold for 2 seconds)
1 rep ½ up (hold for 3 seconds)
1 rep ½ up (hold for 4 seconds)
1 rep ½ up (hold for 5 seconds)
1 full rep
+
1 rep ½ down (holding weight in the half position for 1 second)
1 rep ½ down (hold for 2 seconds)
1 rep ½ down (hold for 3 seconds)
1 rep ½ down (hold for 4 seconds)
1 rep ½ down (hold for 5 seconds)
5 full reps   □

FINISH

WEEK 8 – SATURDAY

(Tick the box when you've completed the relevant exercise)

(a) Warm up options
(Choose one type of warm up, preferably different from the previous day)   □

30 seconds pause

(b) Lower back and buttocks training
1   *Ascending Iso-Matrix Floor Hyperextensions or Prone Lift of legs*
    5 full reps
    1 rep ½ up (holding weight in the half position for 1 second)
    1 rep ½ up (hold for 2 seconds)
    1 rep ½ up (hold for 3 seconds)
    1 rep ½ up (hold for 4 seconds)
    1 rep ½ up (hold for 5 seconds)
    1 full rep
    +
    1 rep ½ down (holding weight in the half position for 1 second)
    1 rep ½ down (hold for 2 seconds)
    1 rep ½ down (hold for 3 seconds)
    1 rep ½ down (hold for 4 seconds)
    1 rep ½ down (hold for 5 seconds)
    5 full reps   □

30 seconds pause

2   *Ascending Iso-Matrix Floor Hyperextensions or Prone Lift of head*
    5 full reps
    1 rep ½ up (holding weight in the half position for 1 second)
    1 rep ½ up (hold for 2 seconds)
    1 rep ½ up (hold for 3 seconds)
    1 rep ½ up (hold for 4 seconds)
    1 rep ½ up (hold for 5 seconds)
    1 full rep
    +
    1 rep ½ down (holding weight in the half position for 1 second)
    1 rep ½ down (hold for 2 seconds)
    1 rep ½ down (hold for 3 seconds)
    1 rep ½ down (hold for 4 seconds)
    1 rep ½ down (hold for 5 seconds)
    5 full reps   ☐

Rest one minute

(c) Thighs and buttocks training
1   *Ascending Iso-Matrix Rear Squats* (with or without weight)
    5 full reps
    1 rep ½ up (holding weight in the half position for 1 second)
    1 rep ½ up (hold for 2 seconds)
    1 rep ½ up (hold for 3 seconds)
    1 rep ½ up (hold for 4 seconds)
    1 rep ½ up (hold for 5 seconds)
    1 full rep
    +
    1 rep ½ down (holding weight in the half position for 1 second)
    1 rep ½ down (hold for 2 seconds)
    1 rep ½ down (hold for 3 seconds)
    1 rep ½ down (hold for 4 seconds)
    1 rep ½ down (hold for 5 seconds)
    5 full reps   ☐

30 seconds pause

2   *Ascending Iso-Matrix Rear Squats* (with or without weight)
    5 full reps
    1 rep ½ up (holding weight in the half position for 1 second)
    1 rep ½ up (hold for 2 seconds)
    1 rep ½ up (hold for 3 seconds)
    1 rep ½ up (hold for 4 seconds)
    1 rep ½ up (hold for 5 seconds)
    1 full rep
    +
    1 rep ½ down (holding weight in the half position for 1 second)
    1 rep ½ down (hold for 2 seconds)
    1 rep ½ down (hold for 3 seconds)
    1 rep ½ down (hold for 4 seconds)
    1 rep ½ down (hold for 5 seconds)
    5 full reps   □

Rest one minute

(d) Calves Training
1   *Ascending Iso-Matrix Donkey Calf Raises*
    5 full reps
    1 rep ½ up (holding weight in the half position for 1 second)
    1 rep ½ up (hold for 2 seconds)
    1 rep ½ up (hold for 3 seconds)
    1 rep ½ up (hold for 4 seconds)
    1 rep ½ up (hold for 5 seconds)
    1 full rep
    +
    1 rep ½ down (holding weight in the half position for 1 second)
    1 rep ½ down (hold for 2 seconds)
    1 rep ½ down (hold for 3 seconds)
    1 rep ½ down (hold for 4 seconds)
    1 rep ½ down (hold for 5 seconds)
    5 full reps   □

20 seconds pause

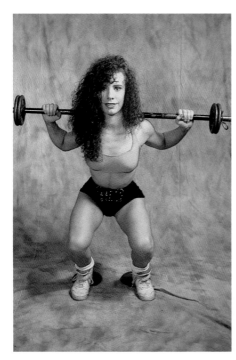

Half-up in the Rear Squat

2   *Ascending Iso-Matrix Donkey Calf Raises*
    5 full reps
    1 rep ½ up (holding weight in the half position for 1 second)
    1 rep ½ up (hold for 2 seconds)
    1 rep ½ up (hold for 3 seconds)
    1 rep ½ up (hold for 4 seconds)
    1 rep ½ up (hold for 5 seconds)
    1 full rep
    +
    1 rep ½ down (holding weight in the half position for 1 second)
    1 rep ½ down (hold for 2 seconds)
    1 rep ½ down (hold for 3 seconds)
    1 rep ½ down (hold for 4 seconds)
    1 rep ½ down (hold for 5 seconds)
    5 full reps   ☐

FINISH

Week 9
The Descending
Iso-Matrix Principle

WEEK 9 – MONDAY

(Tick the box when you've completed the relevant exercise)

(a) Warm up options
Choose one type of warm up (see pages 34–35)   ☐

30 seconds pause

(b) Lower back and buttocks training
1   *Descending Iso-Matrix Floor Hyperextensions or Prone Lift
    of legs*
    5 full reps
    1 rep ½ up (holding weight in the half positon for 5 seconds)
    1 rep ½ up (hold for 4 seconds)
    1 rep ½ up (hold for 3 seconds)
    1 rep ½ up (hold for 2 seconds)
    1 rep ½ up (hold for 1 second)
    1 full rep
    +
    1 rep ½ down (holding weight in the half position for 5
    seconds)
    1 rep ½ down (hold for 4 seconds)
    1 rep ½ down (hold for 3 seconds)
    1 rep ½ down (hold for 2 seconds)
    1 rep ½ down (hold for 1 second)
    5 full reps   ☐

30 seconds pause

2   *Descending Iso-Matrix Floor Hyperextensions or Prone Lift
    of head*
    5 full reps
    1 rep ½ up (holding weight in the half position for 5 seconds)
    1 rep ½ up (hold for 4 seconds)
    1 rep ½ up (hold for 3 seconds)
    1 rep ½ up (hold for 2 seconds)
    1 rep ½ up (hold for 1 second)
    1 full rep
    +
    1 rep ½ down (holding weight in the half position for 5
    seconds)
    1 rep ½ down (hold for 4 seconds)
    1 rep ½ down (hold for 3 seconds)
    1 rep ½ down (hold for 2 seconds)
    1 rep ½ down (hold for 1 second)
    5 full reps   □

Rest one minute

(c) Thighs and buttocks training

1   *Descending Iso-Matrix Rear Squats* (with or without weight)
    5 full reps
    1 rep ½ up (holding weight in the half position for 5 seconds)
    1 rep ½ up (hold for 4 seconds)
    1 rep ½ up (hold for 3 seconds)
    1 rep ½ up (hold for 2 seconds)
    1 rep ½ up (hold for 1 second)
    1 full rep
    +
    1 rep ½ down (holding weight in the half position for 5
    seconds)
    1 rep ½ down (hold for 4 seconds)
    1 rep ½ down (hold for 3 seconds)
    1 rep ½ down (hold for 2 seconds)
    1 rep ½ down (hold for 1 second)
    5 full reps   □

30 seconds pause

2   *Descending Iso-Matrix Rear Squats* (with or without weight)
    5 full reps
    1 rep ½ up (holding weight in the half position for 5 seconds)
    1 rep ½ up (hold for 4 seconds)
    1 rep ½ up (hold for 3 seconds)
    1 rep ½ up (hold for 2 seconds)
    1 rep ½ up (hold for 1 second)
    1 full rep
    +
    1 rep ½ down (holding weight in the half position for 5 seconds)
    1 rep ½ down (hold for 4 seconds)
    1 rep ½ down (hold for 3 seconds)
    1 rep ½ down (hold for 2 seconds)
    1 rep ½ down (hold for 1 second)
    5 full reps   ☐

Rest one minute

(d) Calves Training
1   *Descending Iso-Matrix Donkey Calf Raises*
    5 full reps
    1 rep ½ up (holding weight in the half position for 5 seconds)
    1 rep ½ up (hold for 4 seconds)
    1 rep ½ up (hold for 3 seconds)
    1 rep ½ up (hold for 2 seconds)
    1 rep ½ up (hold for 1 second)
    1 full rep
    +
    1 rep ½ down (holding weight in the half position for 5 seconds)
    1 rep ½ down (hold for 4 seconds)
    1 rep ½ down (hold for 3 seconds)
    1 rep ½ down (hold for 2 seconds)
    1 rep ½ down (hold for 1 second)
    5 full reps   ☐

20 seconds pause

2   *Descending Iso-Matrix Donkey Calf Raises*
    5 full reps
    1 rep ½ up (holding weight in the half position for 5 seconds)
    1 rep ½ up (hold for 4 seconds)
    1 rep ½ up (hold for 3 seconds)
    1 rep ½ up (hold for 2 seconds)
    1 rep ½ up (hold for 1 second)
    1 full rep
    +
    1 rep ½ down (holding weight in the half position for 5 seconds)
    1 rep ½ down (hold for 4 seconds)
    1 rep ½ down (hold for 3 seconds)
    1 rep ½ down (hold for 2 seconds)
    1 rep ½ down (hold for 1 second)
    5 full reps   ☐

FINISH

WEEK 9 – WEDNESDAY

(Tick the box when you've completed the relevant exercise)

(a) Warm Up Options
(Choose one type of warm up, preferably different from the
previous day)   ☐

30 seconds pause

(b) Biceps training

1   *Descending Iso-Matrix Wide Grip Biceps Curls*
    5 full reps
    1 rep ½ up (holding weight in the half position for 5 seconds)
    1 rep ½ up (hold for 4 seconds)
    1 rep ½ up (hold for 3 seconds)
    1 rep ½ up (hold for 2 seconds)
    1 rep ½ up (hold for 1 second)
    1 full rep
    +
    1 rep ½ down (holding weight in the half position for 5 seconds)
    1 rep ½ down (hold for 4 seconds)
    1 rep ½ down (hold for 3 seconds)
    1 rep ½ down (hold for 2 seconds)
    1 rep ½ down (hold for 1 second)
    5 full reps   □

20 seconds pause

2   *Descending Iso-Matrix Narrow Grip Biceps Curls*
    5 full reps
    1 rep ½ up (holding weight in the half position for 5 seconds)
    1 rep ½ up (hold for 4 seconds)
    1 rep ½ up (hold for 3 seconds)
    1 rep ½ up (hold for 2 seconds)
    1 rep ½ up (hold for 1 second)
    1 full rep
    +
    1 rep ½ down (holding weight in the half position for 5 seconds)
    1 rep ½ down (hold for 4 seconds)
    1 rep ½ down (hold for 3 seconds)
    1 rep ½ down (hold for 2 seconds)
    1 rep ½ down (hold for 1 second)
    5 full reps

Rest one minute

(c) *Triceps training*

1   *Descending Iso-Matrix Narrow Grip Lying Triceps Press*
    5 full reps
    1 rep ½ up (holding weight in the half position for 5 seconds)
    1 rep ½ up (hold for 4 seconds)
    1 rep ½ up (hold for 3 seconds)
    1 rep ½ up (hold for 2 seconds)
    1 rep ½ up (hold for 1 second)
    1 full rep
    +
    1 rep ½ down (holding weight in the half position for 5 seconds)
    1 rep ½ down (hold for 4 seconds)
    1 rep ½ down (hold for 3 seconds)
    1 rep ½ down (hold for 2 seconds)
    1 rep ½ down (hold for 1 second)
    5 full reps   ☐

20 seconds pause

2   *Descending Iso-Matrix Medium Grip Lying Triceps Press*
    5 full reps
    1 rep ½ up (holding weight in the half position for 5 seconds)
    1 rep ½ up (hold for 4 seconds)
    1 rep ½ up (hold for 3 seconds)
    1 rep ½ up (hold for 2 seconds)
    1 rep ½ up (hold for 1 second)
    1 full rep
    +
    1 rep ½ down (holding weight in the half position for 5 seconds)
    1 rep ½ down (hold for 4 seconds)
    1 rep ½ down (hold for 3 seconds)
    1 rep ½ down (hold for 2 seconds)
    1 rep ½ down (hold for 1 second)
    5 full reps   ☐

FINISH

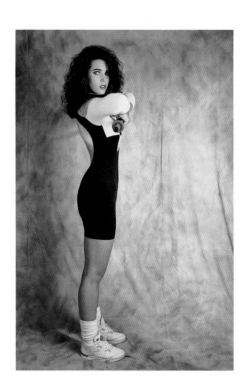

An Upright Row

WEEK 9 – FRIDAY

(Tick the box when you've completed the relevant exercise)

(a) Warm up options
(Choose one type of warm up, preferably different from the
previous day)   ☐

30 seconds pause

(b) Shoulders, triceps and upper back training
1   *Descending Iso-Matrix Upright Rows*
    5 full reps
    1 rep ½ up (holding weight in the half position for 5 seconds)
    1 rep ½ up (hold for 4 seconds)
    1 rep ½ up (hold for 3 seconds)
    1 rep ½ up (hold for 2 seconds)
    1 rep ½ up (hold for 1 second)
    1 full rep
    +

1 rep ½ down (holding weight in the half position for 5 seconds)
1 rep ½ down (hold for 4 seconds)
1 rep ½ down (hold for 3 seconds)
1 rep ½ down (hold for 2 seconds)
1 rep ½ down (hold for 1 second)
5 full reps   ☐

20 seconds pause

2   *Descending Iso-Matrix Lateral Raises*
    5 full reps
    1 rep ½ up (holding weight in the half position for 5 seconds)
    1 rep ½ up (hold for 4 seconds)
    1 rep ½ up (hold for 3 seconds)
    1 rep ½ up (hold for 2 seconds)
    1 rep ½ up (hold for 1 second)
    1 full rep
    +
    1 rep ½ down (holding weight in the half position for 5 seconds)
    1 rep ½ down (hold for 4 seconds)
    1 rep ½ down (hold for 3 seconds)
    1 rep ½ down (hold for 2 seconds)
    1 rep ½ down (hold for 1 second)
    5 full reps   ☐

Rest one minute

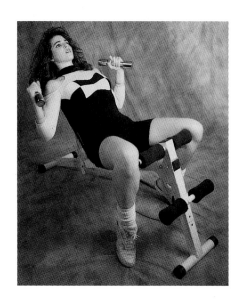

An Incline Bench Press with
dumbbells in the starting
position

(c) Chest, triceps and shoulders training

1 *Descending Iso-Matrix Incline Bench Press*
    (Note: Can be done with dumbbells or a barbell)
    5 full reps
    1 rep ½ up (holding weight in the half position for 5 seconds)
    1 rep ½ up (hold for 4 seconds)
    1 rep ½ up (hold for 3 seconds)
    1 rep ½ up (hold for 2 seconds)
    1 rep ½ up (hold for 1 second)
    1 full rep
    +
    1 rep ½ down (holding weight in the half position for 5
    seconds)
    1 rep ½ down (hold for 4 seconds)
    1 rep ½ down (hold for 3 seconds)
    1 rep ½ down (hold for 2 seconds)
    1 rep ½ down (hold for 1 second)
    5 full reps   □

20 seconds pause

2   *Descending Iso-Matrix Incline Bench Press*
    5 full reps
    1 rep ½ up (holding weight in the half position for 5 seconds)
    1 rep ½ up (hold for 4 seconds)
    1 rep ½ up (hold for 3 seconds)
    1 rep ½ up (hold for 2 seconds)
    1 rep ½ up (hold for 1 second)
    1 full rep
    +
    1 rep ½ down (holding weight in the half position for 5 seconds)
    1 rep ½ down (hold for 4 seconds)
    1 rep ½ down (hold for 3 seconds)
    1 rep ½ down (hold for 2 seconds)
    1 rep ½ down (hold for 1 second)
    5 full reps   ☐

Rest one minute

(d) Midsection training

1   *Descending Iso-Matrix Abdominal Crunch*
    5 full reps
    1 rep ½ up (holding weight in the half position for 5 seconds)
    1 rep ½ up (hold for 4 seconds)
    1 rep ½ up (hold for 3 seconds)
    1 rep ½ up (hold for 2 seconds)
    1 rep ½ up (hold for 1 second)
    1 full rep
    +
    1 rep ½ down (holding weight in the half position for 5 seconds)
    1 rep ½ down (hold for 4 seconds)
    1 rep ½ down (hold for 3 seconds)
    1 rep ½ down (hold for 2 seconds)
    1 rep ½ down (hold for 1 second)
    5 full reps   ☐

20 seconds pause

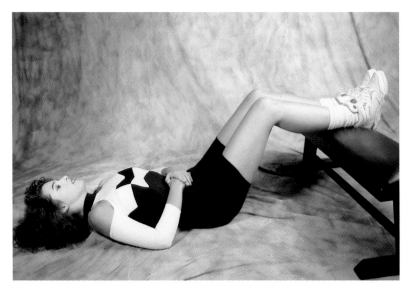

The starting position of the Abdominal Crunch

2   *Descending Iso-Matrix Abdominal Crunch*
   5 full reps
   1 rep ½ up (holding weight in the half position for 5 seconds)
   1 rep ½ up (hold for 4 seconds)
   1 rep ½ up (hold for 3 seconds)
   1 rep ½ up (hold for 2 seconds)
   1 rep ½ up (hold for 1 second)
   1 full rep
   +
   1 rep ½ down (holding weight in the half position for 5 seconds)
   1 rep ½ down (hold for 4 seconds)
   1 rep ½ down (hold for 3 seconds)
   1 rep ½ down (hold for 2 seconds)
   1 rep ½ down (hold for 1 second)
   5 full reps   □

FINISH

Week 10
The Conventional
Iso-Matrix Principle

WEEK 10 – TUESDAY

(Tick the box when you've completed the relevant exercise)

(a) Warm up options
Choose one type of warm up (see pages 34–35) □

30 seconds pause

(b) Shoulders, triceps and upper back training
1 *Conventional Iso-Matrix Roll Press Behind the Neck*
   (Note: A broomstick or hollow length of pipe can be used)
   5 roll presses
   5 ½ up (hold for 5 seconds*)
   5 ½ down (hold 5 seconds)
   5 roll presses
   * For beginners, hold for 3 seconds only □

30 seconds pause

2 *Conventional Iso-Matrix Roll Press Behind the Neck*
   5 roll presses
   5 ½ up (hold for 5 seconds*)
   5 ½ down (hold 5 seconds)
   5 roll presses
   * For beginners, hold for 3 seconds only □

Rest one minute

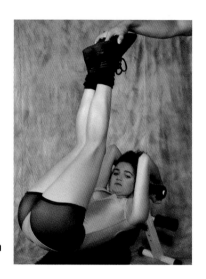

The top position of the Incline Bench
Leg Raise

(c) Chest, triceps and shoulders training

1 *Conventional Iso-Matrix Bench Press*
    5 full reps
    5 ½ up (hold for 5 seconds*)
    5 ½ down (hold 5 seconds)
    5 full reps
    * For beginners, hold for 3 seconds only   ☐

20 seconds pause

2 *Conventional Iso-Matrix Bench Press*
    5 full reps
    5 ½ up (hold for 5 seconds*)
    5 ½ down (hold 5 seconds)
    5 full reps
    * For beginners, hold for 3 seconds only   ☐

Rest one minute

(d) Midsection training

1 *Conventional Iso-Matrix Incline Bench Leg Raises*
    5 full reps
    5 ½ up (hold for 5 seconds*)
    5 ½ down (hold 5 seconds)
    5 full reps
    * For beginners, hold for 3 seconds only   ☐

20 seconds pause

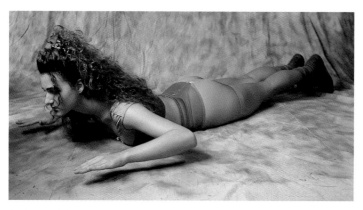

A Prone Lift of the head

2   *Conventional Iso-Matrix Incline Bench Leg Raises*
    5 full reps
    5 ½ up (hold for 5 seconds*)
    5 ½ down (hold 5 seconds)
    5 full reps
    * For beginners, hold for 3 seconds only   ☐

FINISH

WEEK 10 – THURSDAY

(Tick the box when you've completed the relevant exercise)

(a) *Warm up options*
(Choose one type of warm up, preferably different from the
previous day).   ☐

30 seconds pause

(b) *Lower back and buttocks training*
1   *Conventional Iso-Matrix Floor Hyperextensions or Prone Lift
    of legs*
    5 full reps
    5 ½ up (hold for 5 seconds*)
    5 ½ down (hold 5 seconds)
    5 full reps
    * For beginners, hold for 3 seconds only   ☐

30 seconds pause

2   *Conventional Iso-Matrix Floor Hyperextensions or Prone Lift*
    of head
    5 full reps
    5 ½ up (hold for 5 seconds*)
    5 ½ down (hold 5 seconds)
    5 full reps
    * For beginners, hold for 3 seconds only   ☐

Rest one minute

(c) Thighs and buttocks training
1   *Conventional Iso-Matrix Rear Squats*
    5 full reps
    5 ½ up (hold for 5 seconds*)
    5 ½ down (hold 5 seconds)
    5 full reps
    * For beginners, hold for 3 seconds only   ☐

40 seconds pause

2   *Conventional Iso-Matrix Rear Squats*
    5 full reps
    5 ½ up (hold for 5 seconds*)
    5 ½ down (hold 5 seconds)
    5 full reps
    * For beginners, hold for 3 seconds only   ☐

Rest one minute

(d) Calves training
1   *Conventional Iso-Matrix Donkey Calf Raises*
    5 full reps
    5 ½ up (hold for 5 seconds*)
    5 ½ down (hold 5 seconds)
    5 full reps
    * For beginners, hold for 3 seconds only   ☐

30 seconds pause

2   *Conventional Iso-Matrix Donkey Calf Raises*
    5 full reps
    5 ½ up (hold for 5 seconds*)
    5 ½ down (hold 5 seconds)
    5 full reps
    * For beginners, hold for 3 seconds only   ☐

FINISH

WEEK 10 – SATURDAY

(Tick the box when you've completed the relevant exercise)

(a) *Warm up options*
(Choose one type of warm up preferably different from the
previous day)   ☐

30 seconds pause

(b) *Lower back and buttocks training*
1   *Conventional Iso-Matrix Floor Hyperextensions or Prone Lift*
    of legs
    5 full reps
    5 ½ up (hold for 5 seconds*)
    5 ½ down (hold 5 seconds)
    5 full reps
    * For beginners, hold for 3 seconds only   ☐

30 seconds pause

2   *Conventional Iso-Matrix Floor Hyperextensions or Prone Lift*
    of head
    5 full reps
    5 ½ up (hold for 5 seconds*)
    5 ½ down (hold 5 seconds)
    5 full reps
    * For beginners, hold for 3 seconds only   ☐

Rest one minute

(c) Thighs and buttocks training

1   *Conventional Iso-Matrix Rear Squats* (with or without weight)
    5 full reps
    5 ½ up (hold for 5 seconds*)
    5 ½ down (hold 5 seconds)
    5 full reps
    * For beginners, hold for 3 seconds only   ☐

30 seconds pause

2   *Conventional Iso-Matrix Rear Squats* (with or without weight)
    5 full reps
    5 ½ up (hold for 5 seconds*)
    5 ½ down (hold 5 seconds)
    5 full reps
    * For beginners, hold for 3 seconds only   ☐

Rest one minute

(d) Calves training

1   *Conventional Iso-Matrix Donkey Calf Raises*
    5 full reps
    5 ½ up (hold for 5 seconds*)
    5 ½ down (hold 5 seconds)
    5 full reps
    * For beginners, hold for 3 seconds only   ☐

20 seconds pause

2   *Conventional Iso-Matrix Donkey Calf Raises*
    5 full reps
    5 ½ up (hold for 5 seconds*)
    5 ½ down (hold 5 seconds)
    5 full reps
    * For beginners, hold for 3 seconds only   ☐

FINISH

Week 11
The Cumulative
Iso-Matrix Principle

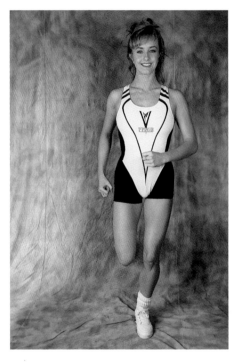

Warming up by running on the spot

WEEK 11 – MONDAY

(Tick the box when you've completed the relevant exercise)

(a) Warm up options
Choose one type of warm up (see pages 34–35) ☐

30 seconds pause

(b) Lower back and buttocks training

1   *Cumulative Iso-Matrix Floor Hyperextensions or Prone Lift
    of legs*
    1 full rep
    1 rep ½ up (hold for 1 second)
    2 reps ½ up (hold for 2 seconds)
    3 reps ½ up (hold for 3 seconds)
    4 reps ½ up (hold for 4 seconds)
    5 full reps
    +
    1 rep ½ down (hold for 1 second)
    2 reps ½ down (hold for 2 seconds)
    3 reps ½ down (hold for 3 seconds)
    4 reps ½ down (hold for 4 seconds)
    5 full reps   □

30 seconds pause

2   *Cumulative Iso-Matrix Floor Hyperextensions or Prone Lift
    of head*
    1 full rep
    1 rep ½ up (hold for 1 second)
    2 reps ½ up (hold for 2 seconds)
    3 reps ½ up (hold for 3 seconds)
    4 reps ½ up (hold for 4 seconds)
    5 full reps
    +
    1 rep ½ down (hold for 1 second)
    2 reps ½ down (hold for 2 seconds)
    3 reps ½ down (hold for 3 seconds)
    4 reps ½ down (hold for 4 seconds)
    5 full reps   □

Rest one minute

(c) Thighs and buttocks training

1   *Cumulative Iso-Matrix Rear Squats* (with or without weight)
1 full rep
1 rep ½ up (hold for 1 second)
2 reps ½ up (hold for 2 seconds)
3 reps ½ up (hold for 3 seconds)
4 reps ½ up (hold for 4 seconds)
5 full reps
+
1 rep ½ down (hold for 1 second)
2 reps ½ down (hold for 2 seconds)
3 reps ½ down (hold for 3 seconds)
4 reps ½ down (hold for 4 seconds)
5 full reps   ☐

30 seconds pause

2   *Cumulative Iso-Matrix Rear Squats* (with or without weight)
1 full rep
1 rep ½ up (hold for 1 second)
2 reps ½ up (hold for 2 seconds)
3 reps ½ up (hold for 3 seconds)
4 reps ½ up (hold for 4 seconds)
5 full reps
+
1 rep ½ down (hold for 1 second)
2 reps ½ down (hold for 2 seconds)
3 reps ½ down (hold for 3 seconds)
4 reps ½ down (hold for 4 seconds)
5 full reps   ☐

Rest one minute

(d) *Calves training*

1   *Cumulative Iso-Matrix Donkey Calf Raises*
     1 full rep
     1 rep ½ up (hold for 1 second)
     2 reps ½ up (hold for 2 seconds)
     3 reps ½ up (hold for 3 seconds)
     4 reps ½ up (hold for 4 seconds)
     5 full reps
     +
     1 rep ½ down (hold for 1 second)
     2 reps ½ down (hold for 2 seconds)
     3 reps ½ down (hold for 3 seconds)
     4 reps ½ down (hold for 4 seconds)
     5 full reps   ☐

20 seconds pause

2   *Cumulative Iso-Matrix Donkey Calf Raises*
     1 full rep
     1 rep ½ up (hold for 1 second)
     2 reps ½ up (hold for 2 seconds)
     3 reps ½ up (hold for 3 seconds)
     4 reps ½ up (hold for 4 seconds)
     5 full reps
     +
     1 rep ½ down (hold for 1 second)
     2 reps ½ down (hold for 2 seconds)
     3 reps ½ down (hold for 3 seconds)
     4 reps ½ down (hold for 4 seconds)
     5 full reps   ☐

FINISH

WEEK 11 – WEDNESDAY

(Tick the box when you've completed the relevant exercise)

(a) *Warm up options*
(Choose one type of warm up, preferably different from the
previous day)   ☐

30 seconds pause

(b) Biceps training

1   *Cumulative Iso-Matrix Wide Grip Biceps Curls*
    1 full rep
    1 rep ½ up (hold for 1 second)
    2 reps ½ up (hold for 2 seconds)
    3 reps ½ up (hold for 3 seconds)
    4 reps ½ up (hold for 4 seconds)
    5 full reps
    +
    1 rep ½ down (hold for 1 second)
    2 reps ½ down (hold for 2 seconds)
    3 reps ½ down (hold for 3 seconds)
    4 reps ½ down (hold for 4 seconds)
    5 full reps   ☐

20 seconds pause

2   *Cumulative Iso-Matrix Narrow Grip Biceps Curls*
    1 full rep
    1 rep ½ up (hold for 1 second)
    2 reps ½ up (hold for 2 seconds)
    3 reps ½ up (hold for 3 seconds)
    4 reps ½ up (hold for 4 seconds)
    5 full reps
    +
    1 rep ½ down (hold for 1 second)
    2 reps ½ down (hold for 2 seconds)
    3 reps ½ down (hold for 3 seconds)
    4 reps ½ down (hold for 4 seconds)
    5 full reps   ☐

Rest one minute

(c) Triceps training

1 *Cumulative Iso-Matrix Narrow Grip Lying Triceps Press*
1 full rep
1 rep ½ up (hold for 1 second)
2 reps ½ up (hold for 2 seconds)
3 reps ½ up (hold for 3 seconds)
4 reps ½ up (hold for 4 seconds)
5 full reps
+
1 rep ½ down (hold for 1 second)
2 reps ½ down (hold for 2 seconds)
3 reps ½ down (hold for 3 seconds)
4 reps ½ down (hold for 4 seconds)
5 full reps   ☐

20 seconds pause

2 *Cumulative Iso-Matrix Medium Grip Lying Triceps Press*
1 full rep
1 rep ½ up (hold for 1 second)
2 reps ½ up (hold for 2 seconds)
3 reps ½ up (hold for 3 seconds)
4 reps ½ up (hold for 4 seconds)
5 full reps
+
1 rep ½ down (hold for 1 second)
2 reps ½ down (hold for 2 seconds)
3 reps ½ down (hold for 3 seconds)
4 reps ½ down (hold for 4 seconds)
5 full reps   ☐

FINISH

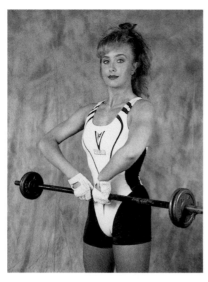

An Upright Row in the half-down position

WEEK 11 – FRIDAY

(Tick the box when you've completed the relevant exercise)

(a) Warm up options
(Choose one type of warm up, preferably different from the previous day)   ☐

30 seconds pause

(b) Shoulders, triceps and upper back training
1   *Cumulative Iso-Matrix Upright Rows*
   1 full rep
   1 rep ½ up (hold for 1 second)
   2 reps ½ up (hold for 2 seconds)
   3 reps ½ up (hold for 3 seconds)
   4 reps ½ up (hold for 4 seconds)
   5 full reps
   +
   1 rep ½ down (hold for 1 second)
   2 reps ½ down (hold for 2 seconds)
   3 reps ½ down (hold for 3 seconds)
   4 reps ½ down (hold for 4 seconds)
   5 full reps   ☐

20 seconds pause

2   *Cumulative Iso-Matrix Lateral Raises*
    1 full rep
    1 rep ½ up (hold for 1 second)
    2 reps ½ up (hold for 2 seconds)
    3 reps ½ up (hold for 3 seconds)
    4 reps ½ up (hold for 4 seconds)
    5 full reps
    +
    1 rep ½ down (hold for 1 second)
    2 reps ½ down (hold for 2 seconds)
    3 reps ½ down (hold for 3 seconds)
    4 reps ½ down (hold for 4 seconds)
    5 full reps   ☐

Rest one minute

(c) Chest, triceps and shoulders training

1   *Cumulative Iso-Matrix Incline Bench Press*
    (Note: Can be done with dumbbells or a barbell)
    1 full rep
    1 rep ½ up (hold for 1 second)
    2 reps ½ up (hold for 2 seconds)
    3 reps ½ up (hold for 3 seconds)
    4 reps ½ up (hold for 4 seconds)
    5 full reps
    +
    1 rep ½ down (hold for 1 second)
    2 reps ½ down (hold for 2 seconds)
    3 reps ½ down (hold for 3 seconds)
    4 reps ½ down (hold for 4 seconds)
    5 full reps   ☐

20 seconds pause

2   *Cumulative Iso-Matrix Incline Bench Press*
    1 full rep
    1 rep ½ up (hold for 1 second)
    2 reps ½ up (hold for 2 seconds)
    3 reps ½ up (hold for 3 seconds)
    4 reps ½ up (hold for 4 seconds)
    5 full reps
    +

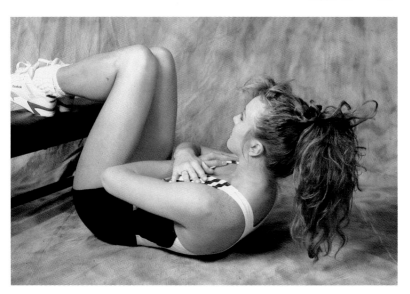

The top position of the Abdominal Crunch

    1 rep ½ down (hold for 1 second)
    2 reps ½ down (hold for 2 seconds)
    3 reps ½ down (hold for 3 seconds)
    4 reps ½ down (hold for 4 seconds)
    5 full reps   □

Rest one minute

(d) Midsection training

1   *Cumulative Iso-Matrix Abdominal Crunch*
    1 full rep
    1 rep ½ up (hold for 1 second)
    2 reps ½ up (hold for 2 seconds)
    3 reps ½ up (hold for 3 seconds)
    4 reps ½ up (hold for 4 seconds)
    5 full reps
    +
    1 rep ½ down (hold for 1 second)
    2 reps ½ down (hold for 2 seconds)
    3 reps ½ down (hold for 3 seconds)
    4 reps ½ down (hold for 4 seconds)
    5 full reps   □

20 seconds pause

2   *Cumulative Iso-Matrix Abdominal Crunch*
     1 full rep
     1 rep ½ up (hold for 1 second)
     2 reps ½ up (hold for 2 seconds)
     3 reps ½ up (hold for 3 seconds)
     4 reps ½ up (hold for 4 seconds)
     5 full reps
     +
     1 rep ½ down (hold for 1 second)
     2 reps ½ down (hold for 2 seconds)
     3 reps ½ down (hold for 3 seconds)
     4 reps ½ down (hold for 4 seconds)
     5 full reps   .□

FINISH

Week 12
The Mixed Iso-Matrix
Principle

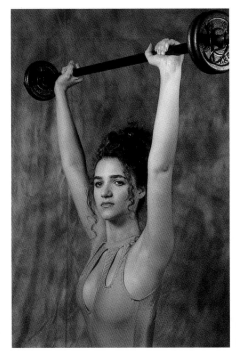

The top position of the Roll
Press

WEEK 12 – TUESDAY

(Tick the box when you've completed the relevant exercise)

(a) Warm up options
Choose one type of warm up (see pages 34–35)   ☐

30 seconds pause

(b) Shoulders, triceps and upper back training

1 *Mixed Iso-Matrix Roll Press Behind the Neck*
    5 roll presses
    3 reps ½ up (hold for 3 seconds)
    3 reps ½ down (no holding)
    3 reps ½ up (no holding)
    3 reps ½ down (hold for 3 seconds)
    5 roll presses   ☐

30 seconds pause

2 *Mixed Iso-Matrix Roll Press Behind the Neck*
    5 roll presses
    3 reps ½ up (hold for 3 seconds)
    3 reps ½ down (no holding)
    3 reps ½ up (no holding)
    3 reps ½ down (hold for 3 seconds)
    5 roll presses   ☐

Rest one minute

(c) Chest, triceps and shoulders training

1 *Mixed Iso-Matrix Bench Press*
    5 full reps
    3 reps ½ up (hold for 3 seconds)
    3 reps ½ down (no holding)
    3 reps ½ up (no holding)
    3 reps ½ down (hold for 3 seconds)
    5 full reps   ☐

20 seconds pause

2 *Mixed Iso-Matrix Bench Press*
    5 full reps
    3 reps ½ up (hold for 3 seconds)
    3 reps ½ down (no holding)
    3 reps ½ up (no holding)
    3 reps ½ down (hold for 3 seconds)
    5 full reps   ☐

Rest one minute

(d) Midsection training

1   *Mixed Iso-Matrix Incline Bench Leg Raises*
    5 full reps
    3 reps ½ up (hold for 3 seconds)
    3 reps ½ down (no holding)
    3 reps ½ up (no holding)
    3 reps ½ down (hold for 3 seconds)
    5 full reps   ☐

20 seconds pause

2   *Mixed Iso-Matrix Incline Bench Leg Raises*
    5 full reps
    3 reps ½ up (hold for 3 seconds)
    3 reps ½ down (no holding)
    3 reps ½ up (no holding)
    3 reps ½ down (hold for 3 seconds)
    5 full reps   ☐

FINISH

WEEK 12 – THURSDAY

(Tick the box when you've completed the relevant exercise)

(a) Warm up options
(Choose one type of warm up, preferably different from the
previous day).   ☐

30 seconds pause

(b) Lower back and buttocks training
1   *Mixed Iso-Matrix Floor Hyperextensions or Prone Lift of legs*
    5 full reps
    3 reps ½ up (hold for 3 seconds)
    3 reps ½ down (no holding)
    3 reps ½ up (no holding)
    3 reps ½ down (hold for 3 seconds)
    5 full reps   ☐

30 seconds pause

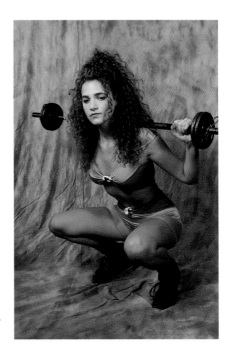

The bottom position of the Rear
Squat

2 *Mixed Iso-Matrix Floor Hyperextensions or Prone Lift of*
   head
   5 full reps
   3 reps ½ up (hold for 3 seconds)
   3 reps ½ down (no holding)
   3 reps ½ up (no holding)
   3 reps ½ down (hold for 3 seconds)
   5 full reps   ☐

Rest one minute

(c) Thighs and buttocks training
1 *Mixed Iso-Matrix Rear Squats*
   5 full reps
   3 reps ½ up (hold for 3 seconds)
   3 reps ½ down (no holding)
   3 reps ½ up (no holding)
   3 reps ½ down (hold for 3 seconds)
   5 full reps   ☐

40 seconds pause

2   *Mixed Iso-Matrix Rear Squats*
    5 full reps
    3 reps ½ up (hold for 3 seconds)
    3 reps ½ down (no holding)
    3 reps ½ up (no holding)
    3 reps ½ down (hold for 3 seconds)
    5 full reps   ☐

Rest one minute

(d) Calves Training
1   *Mixed Iso-Matrix Donkey Calf Raises*
    5 full reps
    3 reps ½ up (hold for 3 seconds)
    3 reps ½ down (no holding)
    3 reps ½ up (no holding)
    3 reps ½ down (hold for 3 seconds)
    5 full reps   ☐

30 seconds pause

2   *Mixed Iso-Matrix Donkey Calf Raises*
    5 full reps
    3 reps ½ up (hold for 3 seconds)
    3 reps ½ down (no holding)
    3 reps ½ up (no holding)
    3 reps ½ down (hold for 3 seconds)
    5 full reps   ☐

FINISH

WEEK 12 – SATURDAY

(Tick the box when you've completed the relevant exercise)

(a) Warm up options
(Choose one type of warm up, preferably different from the
previous day)   ☐

30 seconds pause

(b) Lower back and buttocks training

1 *Mixed Iso-Matrix Floor Hyperextensions or Prone Lift of legs*
   5 full reps
   3 reps ½ up (hold for 3 seconds)
   3 reps ½ down (no holding)
   3 reps ½ up (no holding)
   3 reps ½ down (hold for 3 seconds)
   5 full reps   □

30 seconds pause

2 *Mixed Iso-Matrix Floor Hyperextensions or Prone Lift of head*
   5 full reps
   3 reps ½ up (hold for 3 seconds)
   3 reps ½ down (no holding)
   3 reps ½ up (no holding)
   3 reps ½ down (hold for 3 seconds)
   5 full reps   □

Rest one minute

(c) Thighs and buttocks training

1 *Mixed Iso-Matrix Rear Squats* (with or without weight)
   5 full reps
   3 reps ½ up (hold for 3 seconds)
   3 reps ½ down (no holding)
   3 reps ½ up (no holding)
   3 reps ½ down (hold for 3 seconds)
   5 full reps   □

30 seconds pause

2 *Mixed Iso-Matrix Rear Squats* (with or without weight)
   5 full reps
   3 reps ½ up (hold for 3 seconds)
   3 reps ½ down (no holding)
   3 reps ½ up (no holding)
   3 reps ½ down (hold for 3 seconds)
   5 full reps   □

Rest one minute

(d) Calves training

1. *Mixed Iso-Matrix Donkey Calf Raises*
    5 full reps
    3 reps ½ up (hold for 3 seconds)
    3 reps ½ down (no holding)
    3 reps ½ up (no holding)
    3 reps ½ down (hold for 3 seconds)
    5 full reps   ☐

20 seconds pause

2. *Mixed Iso-Matrix Donkey Calf Raises*
    5 full reps
    3 reps ½ up (hold for 3 seconds)
    3 reps ½ down (no holding)
    3 reps ½ up (no holding)
    3 reps ½ down (hold for 3 seconds)
    5 full reps   ☐

FINISH

Supplementary exercises

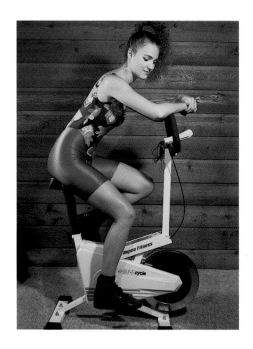

The stationary bike tests your aerobic fitness and exercises your lower legs.

For those trainers who want to make their way to the gym, the Twelve Weeks Matrix Program may be supplemented by substituting any of the following gym-apparatus exercises for the home exercises set out in the routines.

(a) Chest Training Gym Exercises
1   Pec Deck
2   Dips
3   Cable Crossovers

(b) Thigh Training Gym Exercises
    1   Leg Presses
    2   Leg Extensions
    3   Leg Curls
    4   Hack Machine
    5   Inner and Outer Thigh Stretch
    6   Lunges

(c) Biceps
    1   Preacher Bench Curls
    2   Cable Machine Curls

(d) Triceps
    1   Triceps Pushdowns on the Lat Machines

(e) Calves
    1   Seated Calf Raises
    2   Hack Machine Calf Raises

(f) Upper Back
    1   Lat Machine Pulldowns
    2   Seated Cable Rows
    3   Bentover Machine Rows
    4   High Bar Chin Ups

Appendix:
Diet and nutrition—
bodyshaping weight
loss trial

The 'Twelve Weeks to a Better Body' Matrix Program presented in this book can be accompanied by almost any diet which offers a sensible approach to weight management. It is clear that starvation diets are incapable of providing the dietary control necessary for permanent weight reduction. Although crash diets of outlandishly low calorie (or kilojoule) intake may bring about rapid losses in weight, virtually all subjects who lose weight in this way gain it back within six months. More importantly, starvation diets take a great toll on health and happiness. Nutritional deprivation for extended periods can lead to illness and frustration—a total effort all the more frustrating when dieters find themselves regaining all those kilos they worked slavishly to lose.

The Twelve Weeks Matrix Weight Reduction Program emphasises the importance of diet, coupled with the revolutionary step-by-step exercise system presented here. The behavioural changes associated with a healthy lifestyle must also be considered, if long-term results are to be achieved. In this regard the book *101 Vital Tips for a Healthy Lifestyle* (R.S. Laura and J.F. Ashton; HarperCollins, 1993) will provide an extremely helpful companion to this book.

There are two other important points which will help you understand the pattern of the diet you are about to undertake. First, we accept the theory that there is a weight called *Setpoint*, peculiar to every person and below which the metabolic or calorie-burning mechanisms of the body make it difficult to go, regardless of your calorie intake. Fortunately, it is possible to vary calorie levels and the kinds of food ingested in such a way that your Setpoint Weight can be manipulated. You may always have a Setpoint, but with exercise *and* proper diet it is possible to pitch it lower and lower.

Second, we believe that, as long as you consume a lowfat diet

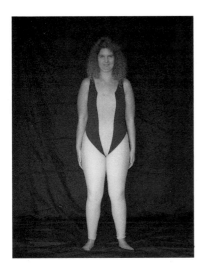 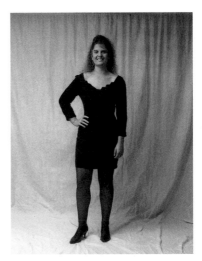

Kim Chuter lost 21 centimetres off her hips in twelve weeks.

about 90 per cent of the time, it is possible occasionally to indulge (not binge) by treating yourself to a craving you may have for some fatty food or other. Dieting is much easier if you can depart every now and then from the tedious rigidity it requires. There is another reason why a carefully placed 'naughty meal' can play a role in an effective weight-loss program. This is that control of weight depends less upon the amount of fatty foods eaten in one meal than it does upon the amount of fatty or high calorie foods you eat *averaged over a week*. Being careful about what you eat *most* of the time, you can afford to eat virtually whatever you want *some* of the time.

Any of a number of approved weight-loss products may be used to good effect while undertaking the 'Twelve Weeks to a Better Body' Matrix Program. However, the before-and-after photos of the subjects shown here reflect the results of the Bodyshaper Trial conducted by Professor Laura, in which each of the subjects shown, while following the Twelve Weeks Matrix Program, substituted one meal each day with the weight-loss product called Firmaloss.

The three individuals involved in the trial all suffered from chronic obesity, and each of them had previously attempted other weight-loss programs without success. In addition to the exercise program set out in this book, each of the subjects was supplied with a '5 Minute Body Shaper' exercise plus sufficient Firmaloss meal-replacement powder for the twelve-week period—on the basis of replacing one meal per day. Each subject was required to visit the Human Performance

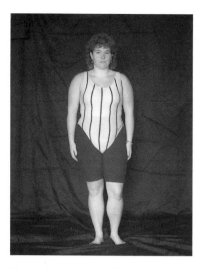 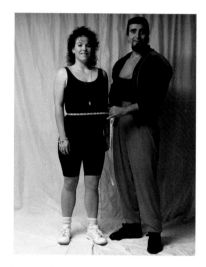

Tania Shotton lost 22 kilograms in twelve weeks.

Research Centre once per week to undertake a Matrix training session under the direction of Professor Laura. Bodyweight and relevant bodyfat measurements were taken at the outset of the session, and time was set aside in every session for discussion of diet and general questions regarding nutrition.

WEIGHT LOSS WITHOUT STARVATION DIETS

The subjects in the trial were permitted to eat as much food as they required to feel satisfied, but they were permitted to eat only whole and fresh foods. One meal every second day could be drawn from the meat group (e.g. fish, chicken, turkey, trim lamb or steak), but all meats were to be prepared by being grilled, baked or steamed. Canned tuna fish and salmon were allowed, but only those packed in water. Fresh vegetables of all kinds were permitted and subjects were encouraged to snack, if necessary, on celery, rock melons, carrot sticks, raw cauliflower and (especially) fresh fruits. The subjects were also requested to minimise the intake of dried fruits for the twelve-week period. The only exception to this rule was the occasional use of a tablespoon of sultanas on breakfast cereal as a sweetener—instead of sugar which was banned, as were white breads, butter, margarine and hard cheeses. Dairy products permitted were those low in fat such as skim milk or lowfat milk. Natural yoghurt, ricotta cheese, fetta cheese and other lowfat cheeses were permitted, along with free-range or vegetarian-source eggs that are now available. Sea-salt, vegetable bouillon, fresh herbs such as basil, oregano, rosemary, marjoram, coriander, ginger, mint and cloves were all recommended as useful seasonings, along with an occasional drop or two of pure olive oil and lemon in some salads.

No restrictions were placed on the *amount* or *kind* of whole foods which could be eaten (other than those specified above). The subjects were allowed to snack between meals twice a day or have the Firmaloss drink between meals. The subjects thus ate two meals of their choice each day, replacing the third meal, usually lunch or dinner, with a Firmaloss Shake. The Shake was used most frequently as a substitute for the lunchtime meal, but one subject used Firmaloss to replace her evening meal almost exclusively for the last four weeks of the trial. Whether it was merely coincidental that this subject lost the most weight or whether it was a direct consequence of taking Firmaloss as an *evening* meal replacement is difficult to determine on the basis of the controls employed in the trial. Such a loss is consistent, however, with the hypothesis that the higher the calorie consumption closer to bedtime, the more likely it is that such calories will lead to greater weight gain in the morning.

RESULTS

The recorded weight losses and consequent reduction in body measurements were substantial. Weight losses during the twelve-week period ranged from a maximum loss of 22 kilos in the case of one subject to a minimum reduction of 7 kilos in the case of another. The reduction of body fat and the drop in overall body measurements were nothing less than phenomenal. One of the subjects lost 28 cm (11 in) off her shoulders, 15 cm (6 in) off her thighs, 22 cm (8½ in) off her hips and 25 cm (10 in) off her waist. These are amazing results.

The subjects also all exhibited significant improvement in overall fitness levels, skin tone and self-esteem. Along with the improvement in fitness levels there were gains in strength.

Acknowledgments

The authors wish to express their appreciation to Rebecca Thurlow for most of the photographs that appear in this book. Her care and artistic touch did much to enhance the impact of the photographs. The before and after shots were taken by Kimberley Mann from Picture-This. Sincere thanks are due to Helene Laura, Sharon Laura, Tracey Moonen, Sheridan Baldwin, Melanie McGregor, Tanya Baptista, Jade Bennett and Tania Riley who appear in the photographs. Finally, we express our gratitude to Coral Johnston for the workout gear specially designed for this book. These and other items of exercise and leisure wear are available from the Corston Collection, PO Box 200, Wickham NSW 2293, phone (049) 50-2360, fax (049) 50-2360.